Finding My Father
A Search For the Truth in the Face of Alzheimer's

Holly Gaskin

Holly Gaskin

Copyright © 2011 Holly Gaskin
All rights reserved.
ISBN: 1453899340
ISBN-13: 978-1453899342

Holly Gaskin

Holly Gaskin

DEDICATION

This book is dedicated to Adolph Robert Cordova, Jr., who has always been there for me in his heart, even when we were far apart. I'll never be too old to be Daddy's Little Girl.

Holly Gaskin

CONTENTS

Acknowledgments

	Adolph: a true short story	10
	Prologue	14
1	My Earliest Memories	16
2	A New Dad	21
3	Cards and Calls	25
4	Digging Up the Past	31
5	The Family I Never Knew	36
6	Wyoming	44
7	Chasing Shadows	49
8	Finding Myself	59
9	Man and Wife	66
10	Reunited	71
11	Our Second Boston Trip	80
12	What Next?	90
13	An Unexpected Twist	96
14	Future Unknown	104
15	Photographs	108
16	Expert Interviews	114

Holly Gaskin

Holly Gaskin

ACKNOWLEDGMENTS

My heartfelt thanks is extended to the following individuals for their valuable contributions to this book:

Stanton O. Berg, Diane Carbo, Cheryl Chow, Rodney Richmond, Richard Taylor, and Patricia Wilkinson

Holly Gaskin

Adolph: A True Short Story

The cab whizzed right past the place.

"Stop!" I cried. The knot in my gut tightened.

I watched the speedometer's needle gradually drop to fifteen miles per hour, but the cabbie didn't stop. He stared at me in his rearview mirror.

"Back there." I pointed over my shoulder. The building was now out of sight, obscured by the giant oak trees that lined the road. "That big brick building…"

"That building abandoned," he argued, in a thick accent that I couldn't quite identify. "Old school. They closed. Nobody there."

"No, the building *next* to the school." I clarified, giving him the house number.

No response.

"Please?"

The cabbie sighed and shifted into reverse, driving slowly, illegally backwards, until I said: "Here."

I had my seatbelt off and the door open before he came to a complete stop. I couldn't take another second in the stifling confines of the non-air conditioned taxi. I shoved a wadded-up twenty in the driver's hand as I scrambled out of the back seat, not waiting for my change. He took off with a grateful toot of his horn.

I stood there, glued to the sidewalk, wondering if I 'd left my courage in the back seat. After all the hassle of getting here, I couldn't take a single step. I saw not a single soul, but I imagined there were eyes peeping at me from behind the curtains of the houses across the street. I spotted Neighborhood Watch signs, and wondered if I looked suspicious, loitering there. The July sun was scorching, almost as unbearable as the inside of the taxi. Already, my forehead was covered with a thin sheen of sweat, and the sleeveless cotton shirt I'd worn with capris and sandals seemed like too much clothing. I was growing increasingly uncomfortable, and more unsure of myself by the second. Was I unwise to have come alone? Or at all? In my panicked state, I thought of running after the taxi and instructing the driver to take me back to my hotel.

Then I saw Adolph.

He was sitting on a bench, next to the building's main entrance, watching me. In spite of the ninety-degree heat, he wore a long-sleeved dress shirt, dark slacks and a necktie. I checked my watch. It was a little past noon, when I'd told him I would arrive. I wondered how long he'd been sitting there, waiting for me. An hour? All morning?

Thirty years? I pushed the thought aside. No more guilt trips. I'd come here to put all that behind me.

My hand shook as I unlatched the cast iron gate. I stepped inside, into *his* world.

Adolph rose and came towards me. His face was familiar, yet barely recognizable. His brown eyes were like I remembered, except that the right one now strayed lazily to one side. The smooth, handsome face, I'd memorized from a few cherished photographs, was now slack, creased with the lines of three hard-lived decades. The waves of thick, black hair I'd inherited were now wispy and gray. His once strong shoulders (which had given a certain little pony-tailed girl piggyback rides almost a lifetime ago) were now stooped. His right hand trembled wildly, grasping at the air as if looking for something to steady him. My God, how much time had I wasted?

Standing a few feet apart, taking each other in, we each waited for the other one to speak first. I had dozens of lines I'd mentally written and stashed away for this very moment. Not to mention hundreds of questions. Now I couldn't recall a single one.

Adolph spoke first.

"Howdy," he said, reaching out his hahond.

I took it in both of mine, and held it to my cheek, struggling to fight back my tears.

"Hi Dad," I said.

Finding My Father

Prologue

I was inspired to write the short story, "Adolph," after I was reunited with my father in the summer of 2009. It was the first time I'd seen him in thirty years. Tracking him down had been difficult, because he had been homeless on and off, staying in shelters or sleeping under bridges. While I was relieved to find out that my father is now living in a safe neighborhood in Boston, with food and shelter, I was distressed to learn that my father is in the early stages of Alzheimer's Disease.

I'd known *something* was wrong. The sporadic cards and letters he sent me were written in shaky, crooked handwriting that became more illegible with each new correspondence. I thought that he either had Parkinson's or that he was suffering neurological damage from years of hard drinking. But whenever I asked him about his health, he avoided answering my questions.

I was planning to visit Dad in 2006, but a personal tragedy in December of that year caused me to delay our reunion for almost two years. I now regret that wasted time.

So, how did my father and I get separated in the first place? Read on…

Finding My Father

Chapter 1

My Earliest Memories

I was born on January 31, 1972 in Seattle, Washington. My father, Adolph Robert Cordova, Jr., was working as a cab driver at the time. He and my mother, Lillian, also brought in extra income by managing the apartment building where they lived. Mom was thirty and my father was thirty-one when they became first-time parents to me, Holly Elizabeth Cordova, their only child.

Eventually, my mother got homesick for her native Long Island and talked my father into moving back there. They did not fly, but drove the more than 2,000 miles to their destination, stopping in my father's home town of Rock Springs, Wyoming on the way, to introduce me to his family. I was only about a year old and don't remember meeting them that first time, but I remember seeing pictures of one of my aunts holding me. I was bawling my eyes out in the photograph and apparently trying to squirm out of her arms!

The three of us moved into a little apartment on Front Street in Greenport. My very first memories are there. I remember Dad going to work at the oyster plant in town, while my mother stayed home to take care of me. I can still remember the layout of the house, the mobile that hung over my crib, and the few, second-hand toys that I had (we were pretty poor). I recall how happy I was when I was allowed to sleep between Mommy and Daddy. I would giggle at how loud he snored, even though it drove my mother nuts! My young life was filled with Daddy's piggyback rides, Mommy's lullabies and happy trips to a downtown pizza place called Fabrizio's.

I also remember my parents fighting. One particular incident stands out in my mind. We were always struggling to make ends meet. When my dad came home one day with a brown paper grocery bag in hand, my mother got excited, because we were almost out of food, and she assumed he'd stopped at the IGA for groceries. When she saw that all that was in the bag was a six-pack of beer and a few pieces of Bazooka bubble gum for me, she hit the roof!

My parents divorced when I wasn't quite three years old. My mother always told me that her reason for leaving was because my father "only worked when he felt like it," and that he drank too much. He stayed in Greenport, while my mother and I moved into a string of rented apartments, before settling in a single-wide trailer in the tiny hamlet of Laurel. Mom opted not to work, choosing instead to dedicate all her time to raising me. Because of this, we had to go on Welfare and use food stamps.

From the time I was four, through when I was six or seven years old, my father visited me regularly. He'd either pick me up at the trailer, or at my grandparents' house in Mattituck, the next town over. He and I would walk downtown, where the Main Street is called Love Lane. My favorite place to visit was a little store called Tic-Tac-Toys. I loved to look at the stuffed animals and tea sets, and my father liked to flirt with Susan, the store owner, who had long red hair and glasses. She could draw any cartoon character you could think of, and her artwork was hung all over the store. She knew my favorite was Woody Woodpecker, and one day, she gave me a hand-drawn picture of the famous, funny bird, which I kept for years. I fell in love with one particular toy in Susan's store; a fuzzy little lamb with a music box inside. I wound up the key and was enthralled when it played "Mary Had a Little Lamb," while his head moved slowly back and forth. I wanted it so badly, but my Dad was just as poor as Mom and I. But when he saw how much my heart was set on that toy, he put it on layaway. I was so happy when I finally was able to bring my little lamb home!

Other times, Dad would take me to Magic Fountain for ice cream, usually soft vanilla in a Dixie cup. The only time I ever remember him yelling at me, was when I didn't feel like finishing it, and I threw the rest of it down the gutter behind his back. He scolded me for wasting money. Other than that, my father was always happy-go-lucky, and fun to be around, kind of like a big kid. He took me to the playground at the beach, where he'd push me on the swings or watch me go up and down the slide. He made me giggle with silly jokes, tried (unsuccessfully) to teach me to tie my shoes, and even taught me to skip. Dad liked to sing a lot, and he sort of played guitar… well, just strummed the instrument, to be more accurate. I have two baby pictures of me in my high chair, laughing with delight as Dad played his guitar for me. He wrote a simple tune for me that went: "Holly Elizabeth, Dad loves you such a lot, He gives you all he's got, Holly Elizabeth." The second verse declared that Mom loved me, and the closing verse assured me God loved me, as well.

Although I was never prevented from seeing my father, from the time of the breakup, I was already being brainwashed against him. I always heard my mother and maternal grandmother refer to him as "Bob," so I started calling him Bob instead of Daddy. Their other nickname for him was "Dopey." You can probably guess what happened. My father was not thrilled when I called him "Dopey," innocently, of course, as though it were any other nickname.

My mother's dad, my Grandpa Newalis, didn't like my father at all. From the onset of the marriage, (as with most of Mom's other boyfriends), Grandpa didn't want to give him a chance. Once Mom and Dad were divorced, Grandpa didn't want Bob in his house. If my father was picking me up at my grandparents' house, I'd have to wait on the porch for Bob to pull up in his Volkswagen Beetle. Then I'd get the go-ahead to go outside to meet him.

Mom starting dating again as soon as she was single. She had a string of boyfriends. There was Billy, who was tall, blond and handsome. He put together a toy box for me one Christmas. But he lived all the way in Queens, about seventy-five miles away, and Mom didn't even have a car. Ronnie was another nice boyfriend. He drove a van with a CB radio in it. (This WAS the 1970s, remember!) He let me talk on it. The "handle" he gave me was "Cupcake." Another of my mom's beaus was named K.C. (or was it Casey?). He was worth some big bucks. I believe he owned a commercial ice machine company. I'd never been in such a big house before! There was an older guy Mom dated, named Bob White, like the bird. He was friendly towards me. The only man Mom dated who I didn't like was Stash. I could tell he didn't really want anything to do with me, either. He had a son who did nothing but bang on a drum set the whole time Mom and I were at their house, until my mother complained she had a headache and we left.

During this time, I only remember my father having one girlfriend. Her name was Lesley. She had brown hair, cut in a Dorothy Hamill 'do, and great big glasses. She was a nice lady, who laughed a lot.

Dad disappeared from the picture around the time my mother became involved with a man named Bud Olmsted. Bud was seventeen years older than mom, a widower with a teenage daughter. When he and Mom got engaged, I was happy and excited. I liked Bud a lot at the time.

I'm not sure if my father's leaving had to do with this turn of events. Maybe he thought he was being replaced. He wound up moving to Boston, where he resumed his career as a cab driver. I don't even remember him saying goodbye to me, or how the news was broken to me that he was moving far, far away. I do remember missing him. I didn't talk about it, though. Even though I only was six or seven years old, I knew that my father was a taboo topic. Whenever his name was spoken, it was with angry connotations, either because of something he'd done in the past, or because he'd fallen behind on child support payments.

One day, I was so sad about the whole situation, that I started crying uncontrollably, out of the blue. My mother asked me what was wrong, trying to comfort me, but I only cried harder.

Through my sobs, I told her: "You'll get mad at me if I tell you."

"No I won't. I promise," she said.

After some hesitation I confessed: "I miss Bob."

"WHAT?!?" she screamed. Her face turned red with rage. I thought she was going to hit me.

"You promised you wouldn't yell!" I blubbered.

"Well, I never thought you'd say anything like THAT!" she screamed at me.

And so I learned not to bring up my father anymore.

Chapter 2

A New Dad

My mother and Bud were married in 1979, when I was seven years old and in the second grade. Bud was a funny guy, with what my mom described as a "dry sense of humor." They had met in a bar. Like my real father, my stepdad drank a lot. Unlike my dad, however, Bud was able to hold his liquor, and also hold down a good job, as a fire inspector. Every evening, after supper, he'd make himself a screwdriver and sit down to watch TV. When the glass was empty, he'd mix himself another and watch more TV, repeating the process until he eventually fell asleep in his chair.

This marriage started off on a high note, but pretty soon, all the shiny newness began to wear off. For all his witticisms and kindness, Bud had a mean streak as well. He liked to get my mother drunk as comic entertainment for his drinking buddies from the fire department. I know this because they took me to the bars with them! I drank Shirley Temples while they drank screwdrivers. (To this day, that is the one mixed drink I refuse to take even a sip of.)

When I was seven or eight, I had one of the most frightening experiences of my childhood. It was nighttime, and the three of us were heading home from one of their favorite bars, either the Blue Top or the Broken-Down Valise. Mom was at the wheel, and Bud was in the passenger seat. Both were inebriated, but Mom much more so than Bud. He was able to handle a few drinks and still be as coherent as when he was sober; you wouldn't know he'd been drinking unless you'd seen him with the glass in his hand. My mother, on the other hand, seemed to get three times as drunk as Bud on the same amount of alcohol. To him, this was a farce. She'd get so intoxicated that she made an embarrassing spectacle of herself. On this particular night, she was so drunk, that she was convinced she'd left Bud behind at the bar, when he was sitting right beside her! She kept trying to make a U-turn right in the middle of Route 25. Bud was laughing hysterically and kept jerking the steering wheel to try to stop her from turning around. I was shaking, terrified, in the back seat, positive that we were going to get in an accident. Finally, Bud got her to realize that he was right there in the car with her, not back at the bar, and God got us home safely.

During the four years that Bud and my mother were married, I did not hear from my father at all. I don't know whether he stopped trying to communicate with me, or if his cards and phone calls were ignored and never mentioned to me. Also, there was the fact that we moved a few times, so it would have been hard for Dad to track me down. (He still had my grandparent's phone number, but they weren't about to give him any information.)

The November I was in third grade, we sold our little log cabin in Mattituck and moved to East Quogue, in the Hamptons, so Bud wouldn't have as far as a commute to work. We rented a beautiful, two story home for a few months, but we couldn't afford to buy it. We finally bought and settled into a small green ranch house, on a dirt road that wasn't even on the map.

Not long after they said their vows, Mom and Bud's marriage started to turn rocky. A big factor in this was Bud's teenage daughter from his first marriage, Christine. She hated my mother. The feeling was mutual. She and Christine were always at each other's throats. A classic "troubled teen," Christine was often in "reform school" more often than she was home with us. The so-called "school" was actually an institution for teens with disciplinary problems. When she came home to live with us, there was usually chaos. Either she was trying to pick a fight with my mother, or sneaking boys over when Mom and Bud weren't at home. She was generally nice to me, but she was very jealous. She was the very definition of a "Daddy's Girl," and she resented my mother and I for coming between them. I felt bad, because I wanted to have a big sister to hang out with. I only called Bud "Dad" a few times. Christine overheard me once and had a fit. From then on, I just called him Bud.

Bud was very controlling. He wouldn't let my mother work, and only gave her a weekly allowance, as if she were a little kid who'd done all her chores. He referred to her as "The Little Woman" when he introduced her to his friends. Bud's words were his weapons; he only physically punished me once, for nor eating. That one time, however, was enough to make me so afraid of him that I could barely talk when he was in the same room. If I had anything to say to my mother, I'd whisper it in her ear. This irked Bud, because he presumed I was talking about him.

At times, Bud did make an effort to be a dad. He taught me how to ride a two-wheeler. He made a couple of attempts to buy my affection with animals, bringing home a parakeet when I was in second grade, and a Siberian Husky puppy named Tasha when I was in fourth. As it happened, the bird, Sylvester, wound up being my mom's pride and joy, and the dog became totally imprinted on Bud. What I really wanted was a kitten, but Bud hated cats. In fact, he bragged to my mother about how he'd once taken a litter of kittens that he found on his property, put them in a bag with some heavy rocks, and dumped the in Long Island Sound to drown them! My mother and I were shocked. Mom remarked to me that she never knew Bud had such a "cruel streak," and ruefully reflecting that "you never really know someone until you live with them."

Although Bud would occasionally help me with a science project, or ask how I was doing in school, he was pretty much uninterested in my school activities. Mom managed to drag him to my third grade talent show, but that was it. He never came to any of my spring concerts, chorus performances or school plays, and Mom was too embarrassed to attend them alone. She'd drop me off at the school and I would get a ride home with a friend. Thinking back on this today, I wish I at least had video tapes of those occasions to share with my father, to show him some of the moments that he missed. If only he hadn't moved to Boston, I think he would have come to every single one of those events.

The stricter Bud got with me (mostly about my being such a picky eater), and the meaner he was towards my mom, the more I missed my real father. Of course, I was still fearful of bringing up the topic, given my mother's reaction years before. My emotions built up like a balloon filling with water, and one day, while Bud was at work, I finally burst. Through tears, I confessed to Mom how much I still missed Bob. This time, my mother was sympathetic, and her eyes were soon brimming with tears, too. When I told her I was so afraid of upsetting her, that I was afraid to even say the name "Bob," even if I was talking about Bob Barker from "The Price Is Right," she cried and kept apologizing for the past. What a load off my chest!

Finally, when I was eleven, my mother got sick of Bud's drinking and his temper, and of Christine's meddling. She left him, and we moved into her parents' house. I was relieved. My only regret was that I never got to say goodbye to my friends in East Quogue School.

My father somehow found out about this (probably because he got a notification that he had to resume making child support payments). He began sending me cards on holidays and even phoned from time to time. Ideally, we should have started rebuilding our relationship then, but things were not that simple.

Chapter 3

Cards and Calls

I had heard lots of horror stories from my mother about her childhood. Her father had physically abused her and her brother (my Uncle Bill) throughout their entire childhoods. "He beat us with a leather strap 'til we were black and blue," she told me many times. When Uncle Bill was in his mid-teens, he kept getting in trouble with the law (drugs, stealing and crashing a car, you name it) and Grandpa kicked him out of the house. Forever. Even though Uncle Bill straightened out his life, got married and had two sons of his own, Grandpa never forgave him. It was really hard on my grandmother, because Uncle Bill sent her letters and photographs of his adorable boys, Jesse and Zac, and she wanted so much to hold her grandbabies and smother them with kisses! Instead, she kept their pictures inside an old pocketbook, well-hidden in a corner of her closet. Grandpa couldn't find out they were in touch, or he'd have a fit.

When I was very little, my great-grandmother, whom I called "Granny," lived with Grandma and Grandpa. She was my grandmother's mother, a sweet lady who liked to crochet and who always made a fuss over me. I remember she always had rolls of Tums (OTC heartburn medication) all over the house. When I was four, we found out that her chronic bellyaches were due to stomach cancer. It was too late to do anything about it. When he heard the news, my grandfather threw her out of the house! I don't know if he was superstitious about sickness, or if he was just plain mean. Granny moved in with my mother and me in our little, single-wide trailer. She slept ion my bed and I slept with Mommy in hers. Mom took care of her until she got so ill that she had to be admitted to the hospital. I'd accompany Mom and Grandma when they visited her, but I had to wait in the lobby, because I was too young to go up to her room. Grandpa never once visited her while she was there. It's like he was mad at her for getting ill! She died a week or so after we brought her in.

Given Grandpa's history, I'm sure that choosing to move back in with him was a dead-end last resort for Mom. Prior to living under his roof, I had never personally been the target of Grandpa's rage. He always called me his little "Punkin'," and we did a lot of fun things together, like fishing, working in the garden or reading the "funny sheets" together. When I was small, he did things with me that a dad would've done. I could hardly believe that this was the same monster who regularly beaten his children and his wife thirty-some years ago.

I always knew he had a bad temper, though. Mom and Grandma would worriedly watch the calendar for Full Moons, because that's when Grandpa tended to explode. He'd start out being unusually quiet, silently brooding, until he found something to blow up about; whether it was dirty dishes in the sink, Grandma overcooking or undercooking something for dinner, me talking too long on the phone or if my mother stayed out too late with her friends. Maybe it was our fault if the sky wasn't blue enough that day. It could be any little thing to send him into a tirade. When the crap hit the fan, Grandpa would stomp in and out of the room, yelling at us in a booming voice, calling us names and slamming doors. These episodes could last a few minutes, or drag out for an hour. He'd storm out of the house. *Slam!* A minute later, he'd come charging back in, to shout something he'd forgotten to say, or needed to say again. Then, back outside. *Slam!* If we were lucky, he'd take off in his blue Toyota pickup once he was finished, to go for a ride to cool his head. It gave us a chance to breathe and recollect our wits. When he returned, he'd give us the silent treatment, not speaking to us at all for a day or two. The phrase "walking on eggshells" could have been invented for my mom, grandmother and me.

Grandpa had not only disliked my father; Mom told me that he'd never liked *any* of her boyfriends except Bud. (Figures!) He blamed my mother for the breakup of that marriage and continually "rubbed her nose in it." While Grandpa never actually forbade me from having contact with my dad, it was an unspoken rule. The attitude I picked up from him was "why would you *want* to?"

Finding My Father

My father addressed all correspondence to me: Holly Cordova, c/o Beatrice Newalis, my grandmother. He knew better than to put his name or return address on the envelope, but I'm sure the Boston postmark must have raised a question mark in Grandpa's mind. In site of sneaking the letters past Grandpa, I still had no privacy when it came to Dad's correspondence. My mother would insist on reading his cards and letters. "What's he say? What'd he write?" she'd press. I had no choice but to hand them over to her. She and my grandmother would make fun of whatever he'd written, laughing at him and remarking how "stupid" and "dopey" he was. Sometimes they'd talk me into ripping up the cards and throwing them away, but I kept most of them.

Some of the messages he scrawled in his messy penmanship were a bit weird. Stuff like: *"Always remember you're American first (by birth). Just about everybody in America is of mixed nationality."* That unusual message came in a Valentines Day card. He ended his note with a sentiment that was easier to understand: *"I love you, and I miss you."* I lost the envelope for that card, so I'm not sure of the year I received it. In another, from Valentines Day of 1985, my father declared that he was trying to get a car to come see me. This scared the crap out of me, to be honest. I was afraid he was going to show up and kidnap me!

My Dad liked to jot brief messages to me inside greeting cards that did most of the talking for him. That's why I was so surprised to receive a full-page letter from him in January of 1984.

Dear Holly,

Just a few lines to let you know I'm thinking of you. I heard you like to write books. That's good. I hope someday you have a bestseller.

I'm working, it's snowing and my feet are wet. But that's par for the course.

You probably have a lot of questions that need answering about me and your mother and why we divorced. I realize it must have been terribly hard on you. I hope someday you'll understand what took place. As for me, I love you and nothing will ever change that.

Hope to see you soon! I'll send you something for your birthday.

Love,
Dad

The Christmas when I was thirteen, Dad sent me a greeting card with a fifty dollar bill in it. Mom and Grandma were shocked, wondering out loud where he could have gotten it. For once, they had nothing bad to say about him. Me, being a pre-teen in the mid-1980s, he might as well have sent me a thousand bucks!

The most uncomfortable times were when my father actually tried to call me. I was never allowed any privacy during the five years I lived in that house. The only telephone, an old, beige, rotary model, was in the dining room, which opened right up into the living room, with no door in between The rooms were small, and there was not enough space for secrets. A whisper in the kitchen, it seemed, could carry all the way to the front porch.

On the rare occasions when Dad called, I'd be surrounded by prying ears. Mom and Grandma were usually sitting at the dining room table, Grandma playing solitaire and Mom doing word search puzzles. Grandpa, would be seated in his armchair in the living room with his feet up on a hassock, watching television. I was the proverbial "monkey in the middle," stuck between both eavesdropping teams. I'd keep my back to them and my voice low as possible, but it didn't matter. Grandpa would turn the volume down whenever I was on the phone, presumably so that I could hear better. Of course, his true motive was to be able to hear *me* better. I was always super-nervous when I was on the phone with my dad (or even with school friends), because I was conscious that I was being watched and listened to. I felt like I was in a goldfish bowl. I would answer my father's questions in emotionless, one-word responses, never offering any extra information of my own.

"So, you write books now?" he asked me.

"Yeah," I said. I couldn't bring myself to elaborate.

"Are you doing good in school?"

"Uh-huh," I'd reply, but I couldn't tell him about my teacher, my friends or boys that I liked. Grandpa was always sitting right there, with his ears pricked, trying to pick up clues on who I might be talking to. I'm glad we didn't have another extension in the house, or he would've been on it, ordering me to hang up and probably hurling some choice four-letter words at my dad.

Adding to the anxiety surrounding the topic of my father, was the fact that anytime I misbehaved, my mother and grandmother would threaten to send me to live with him. This would always send me into tearful hysterics, and they would laugh at me. Looking back on this, I know now that they weren't serious, but as a twelve-year-old, those words put the fear of God in me. I'd already had my family broken apart twice; I didn't want my life to be upended once again.

When I was about thirteen, all correspondence from my father mysteriously died off. At the time, I didn't think too much about it. I thought it would be nice if he sent me fifty bucks again, but that didn't happen. Other than that, my father was a stressful topic, and I didn't complain when the cards and phone calls stopped coming.

After five stressful years in my grandparents' household, my mother and I moved out. I was sixteen. It was a relief to finally be free of the wrath of Grandpa. Mom and I moved into a rented house in a different area of Mattituck. Finally, I was allowed to be a real teenager! Grandpa had never let me have friends over or play loud music or watch MTV. Now I could do all of these things!

By that time, the letters and cards from Dad had long since ceased. The only proof I had that he was still alive were the child support checks Mom received every now and then. The more I matured, the more I realized that I had my own opinions about things, my father included. I didn't hate him. I didn't think he was stupid or dopey. Those were other people's opinions, which had been forced onto me.

I made the decision to try and reestablish contact with my father. My mother had mixed feelings about this. Talk about holding a grudge!

My goal was clear and simple: find out where Dad was living and reach out to him. This, however, would prove more difficult than I ever dreamed it could be.

Chapter 4

Digging Up the Past

In 1991, at age nineteen, I was hospitalized for more than four months in South Oaks Hospital in Amityville, NY suffering from Anorexia Nervosa and Bulimia. I weighed 68 pounds when they checked me in. The medical staff there said it was a miracle I didn't die. I was told that my body was basically feeding on its own muscle tissue to stay alive. If I'd waited much longer, it would have affected my heart. There were myriad factors that led up to my eating disorders, but that would be another book in itself.

During my hospitalization, my father was one of the issues that came up in therapy. In family counseling, my social worker, Paulette, agreed that it would be a positive thing for me to reconnect with Dad. It was decided that I would resume my search for him while I was in the safe, controlled environment of the hospital. That way, if things didn't go well, I'd have a strong support system around me.

I was afraid to broach the topic with my mother. Sometimes I wound up breaking the news to her over the phone. I held my breath, waiting for an explosion. Much to my surprise, my mother didn't get angry. Even though she knew I had entertained the idea of finding him, she misunderstood my intentions. She presumed that I hated him and that I wanted to find him to confront him.

Relieved to have broken the ice, I bombarded her with questions, such as did my father ever remarry? She told me yes, he did, but she didn't know any details. I got very excited at the thought that I might have a half-brother or half-sister somewhere out there. At the same time, I was worried that Dad's new wife might be real possessive and might not want me trying to contact her husband.

I wanted to know if my father had any brothers and sisters, and my mother said yes, he did, quite a few of them. I was amazed to think I had Aunts and Uncles I'd never met, and a new set of grandparents, if they were still living. I laugh now, reading my journal entry from August 12, 1991:

"Bob is probably about 52 now. God, that sounds so old! I'd better hurry up and find him!"

I was still calling my father "Bob" in my journals, not "Dad."

I was almost positive that he'd have an unlisted phone number. But, to my total shock and amazement, I called Boston information and they had a listing for an "A. Cordova." It took me a couple of days to gather the nerve to call the number. I made the call from my social worker's office. I brought along Genny, a friend I'd made in the eating disorders unit, for moral support. As it turned out, the number was not my father's. It belonged to an Andrea Cordova. No relation.

In my next family counseling session, Dad was the main topic of discussion. My mother described him as a "sore subject" with her. Paulette, the social worker, asked why. My mother reluctantly divulged an unsavory slew of facts about his behavior, which she could only describe as "weird." According to her, Bob had warned her and me about using public transportation. He scared me by telling me that someone on the bus might try to kidnap me. Also, he supposedly ordered her not to leave the house when he wasn't home. "And Lord help me if I did," Mom said. She claimed he'd once given her two black eyes "for mentioning guns." I still have trouble believing this. I remember my parents fighting a lot, and my father yelling and cursing at Mom, but I don't recall him ever hitting her. Considering how young I was at the time, it's pretty amazing how many details I can recall from that period of my life. I remember laying in my baby crib, crying because I wanted to sleep between Mommy and Daddy in their big bed. I can still recall all of my stuffed animals and their names: Fido, Toby, Teddy, Freddy and Raggedy Ann. I remember wearing red patent leather shoes, a polka dot dress and a little sailor cap (I cried when mice chewed holes in my hat and it had to be thrown away). If I can remember these mundane things in such detail, you'd think I'd most certainly recall something as traumatic as Daddy giving Mommy two black eyes.

Other revelations: My father had done jail time for robbery. Also, he had some sort of superstition about illness in the family. One of his sisters had given birth to a baby that was mentally retarded, and Bob always refused to talk about it. He wouldn't discuss any sickness in the family.

This hit me hard on many levels. First, would he ever understand or acknowledge my Anorexia and depression? Would he not want to talk about it, or tell me that my problems were all in my head?

Also, I'd been diagnosed at age sixteen with Neurofibromatosis, a genetic disorder which causes benign tumors to grow anywhere on the body at any time. It can also cause learning disabilities, vision and hearing problems, bone deformities, and in rare cases, cancer. I am lucky to have just a mild case, with tell-tale "café au lait" spots and benign fibromas (growths) on my body, mostly in areas covered by clothes. I was thought to have been a "spontaneous mutation." That is, no one else in my family is known to have this condition. But then again, I really didn't know anything about my father's family. Maybe there were other cases of NF among them. But if Dad really saw any kind of sickness as a stigma, I might never get the truth out of him.

Paulette suggested trying to find him through the Child Support Agency. I thought it might be preferable to find out his address and just pop in, unannounced, rather than call or write a letter. That way, if he didn't know I was coming, he wouldn't have a chance to run away from me.

August 16, 1991

I talked to Mom on the phone today. I had asked her to call the child support people and ask them to trace my dad for me. They told her that they can't do that for anybody. I feel like I'm at a dead end. But, I won't give up. I spoke to Paulette about my options. Unfortunately, she's going on vacation for a week.

I can do one of many things... I can get access to a library and look up his phone number in an out-of-state phone book. I can try and find an old card he sent me and get the address from that. I can write to someone like "Dear Abby" and ask what agency might help me. I can try to find one of his brothers or sisters. (Mom doubts that his parents are alive.) Mom's friend, Mabel, dated my dad after he divorced my mom. Maybe she might know something. She and my mom go to Bingo together every Thursday.

This was before the internet was so common. There was no Google and no Facebook, no such thing as finding somebody instantaneously. I wouldn't have been allowed access to the in the strict hospital ward anyway. I was totally dependant on outside sources. Mainly, Mom. And she wavered in her willingness to help me find Dad.

August 28, 1991

Talked to Mom on the phone about my father today. The conversation got pretty hairy. I asked her to call Wyoming information, to see if any of Bob's brothers were still living in Rock Springs. She started making excuses, saying they probably don't live there anymore. Also, she said that Bob didn't want to keep in contact with his family. They probably wouldn't know where he is. I finally convinced her to dial the freakin' number. She called back to say that there was an Alex Cordova in the book, but the number was unlisted. I yelled at her that if he was unlisted, his name wouldn't have been in the f***in' phone book! How stupid does she think I am?!? Mom claims she can't remember if Bob had a brother named Alex or not. I told her to bring me the phone number next time she visits me.

Within a few days, Mom had had a change of heart.

September 4, 1991

Mom brought me a list of phone numbers of Cordovas in Wyoming. And guess what? She RECOGNIZES some of the names on the list as my dad's brothers! MY UNCLES!! The names she didn't recognize, she assumes are Bob's nieces and nephews... MY COUSINS!! She got these from the Riverhead library. I didn't think she'd go through with it. What a shocker!

One number is for an Adolph Cordova. It might be my grandfather. Mom is stunned that he might still be alive. He'd be really old.

I'm going to be making some very scary phone calls soon!

Chapter 5

The Family I Never Knew

I was terrified, making that first phone call. What if they hated my father for deserting them, and thought I was no better than him? I could not have been more wrong.

September 8, 1991

I begged Mom to sit by me while I made the call. I needed her support. I was so scared. I was positive I'd be rejected. Maybe they hate Bob and everyone associated with him. Mom didn't want to be with me. She was like, "I don't want ANYTHING to do with this!" I finally got her to cooperate. I wasn't sure which number to call. I thought of calling his brother, Ernie, one of the ones Mom remembered meeting. Mom said to call the Adolph one. She said that he was probably dead, but that one of the other "kids" (Bob's siblings) is living there. So I dialed that one.

As I listened to the soft, distant ringing of the phone, I wanted to hang up. I sort of wished no one would answer. Someone did. It was my grandmother. She sounded dazed as I explained who I was. "Bob's daughter," I said. "Adolph Jr.'s daughter." Then she began to get very excited. She put her husband, my grandfather, on. He was so deaf he couldn't hear me. His wife took the phone back.

"Do you want to speak with one of my daughters?" she asked.

I told her yes, and found myself speaking to my Aunt Rose. She was blown away that I'd called. Nobody was angry. In fact, just they opposite. They were all happy to hear from me! Rose says the whole family was curious about me all these years.

"I don't think you realize what a big family you have," she said. She told me she had often wondered why I didn't try to make contact with the family. I felt guilty. I guess I never really thought about it

until recently. I didn't even know he had a lot of brothers and sisters. Rose urged me to come to Wyoming sometime soon. She actually lives in Salt Lake City, Utah. She says it's ironic that I called when I did, when she just happened to be visiting her parents.

I asked Rose if my grandfather realized who I was. It was hard for me to tell, with his hearing problem. Rose said yes. She ran and got a picture of me as a baby and showed him, and then he understood. She says she's the only one in the family with a picture of me, and she still shows it to everyone. Holy cow. Really makes me believe in my Higher Power. I just inherited an entire family!

When my grandmother got back on the phone, she was crying.

"Hello, my granddaughter!" she said, in a heavy Spanish accent. She told me she wants me to come see her "before I die." (Mom says they must be in their eighties now.) I wanted to hop on a plane right then and there!

Of course, the original reason I called was to get information on my father. Unfortunately, they haven't heard from him in an even longer time than I have. They don't know if he's alive or dead. I told her I'd last heard from him when I was twelve, that he'd lived in Boston, and that he remarried. She was surprised.

I have wondered sometimes if my father is dead. In a way, that would be easier to accept than knowing he'd been rejecting me all these years, and that he just doesn't love me. (Mom told me later that he can't be dead, because she still receives child support payments every once in a while. I'd forgotten about that.)

Rose says that her mother's dying wish is to see "Junior" again. They have also been frantically searching for him for ages. I'm more determined than ever to find him now! He promised in all those letters long ago, that one day he'd answer all my questions "when I was old enough to understand." He can bet his ass I have plenty of questions! When I find him, I won't know whether to hug him or hit him! My mom gave me the number for the child support agency and the name of his case worker. I'm gonna try to call from Paulette's *office tomorrow. They refused to disclose his whereabouts to my mother. Maybe Paulette can help me get information out of them. I've needed to find him for myself. Now I need to find him for ALL of us.*

My mother was surprised how well everything went. She actually started crying. She was amazed that the family wasn't bitter towards her because of the divorce. They even asked how she was doing. My new grandmother even offered to help out financially if I have a problem getting out there to Wyoming. My mother told me: "She was always such a kindhearted person." I think I already like her better than the grandmother I already have! Is that terrible or what?

Mom tells me how much it snows in Wyoming. She was there once to witness it. It's similar to Minnesota, where her brother lives. I told her I wouldn't mind. For some reason, I was thinking she'd go with me to meet the family. She doesn't want to. What for? I'm so used to her accompanying me everywhere. Maybe it's time I let go of Mommy's hand and crossed the street by myself, so to speak. But it's such a major step to make alone! But I have a feeling that it will be healthy for me. The scariest part will be getting on a plane.

My mom says she didn't remember Rose. She sounds very understanding and intelligent. I bonded with her over the phone, if that's possible. Rose says that her oldest brother, Henry, passed away last year. He was the one closest to Bob. Rose says they were "inseparable." I wonder if my father even knows Henry died...

Ironically, just as my mother had assumed my paternal grandparents had died, my father's family presumed that Dad was deceased.

September 21, 1991

Mom called tonight. She said that my Uncle Alex called her. They talked for half an hour. She told him about my being in the hospital and gave him the number here. He wants to meet me too!

Mom's patient, Billy, died today. (My mother was a home health aide at this time.) *She's now out of a job. She told Uncle Alex about our hard times, and he is sending us $300! I feel funny accepting it from a "stranger." I hope Mom didn't actually ASK for it. I've always thought that the more you suffer in life, the greater your reward will be later on. I'm finally getting my share.*

The following day I "met" my Uncle Alex.

September 22, 1991

I spoke with my Uncle Alex on the phone. He told me to call collect, but I couldn't do that. Alex says that he never thought twice about being generous with his money. He says that you only get one family; the rest is just material.

He asked me: "How long are you going to be in the place you're in (the hospital)?" I told him I didn't know. Probably a few more weeks. He wants me to come visit the family too. He has a daughter my age, 19, named Allie. Alex reiterated what Aunt Rose said about my having a large family. There were 11 brothers and sisters in all, including my father! The oldest died last year, leaving six girls and four boys. ALL of my aunts and uncles had kids... one had 8 or 9!!! Holy cow! I have a lot of cousins, don't I? I suggested maybe visiting around the holidays. Wouldn't it be great to have a family reunion around Christmastime?

I worked hard at getting better, following my nutritional plan and attending all the meetings and group therapy that I was supposed to. When I'd first been admitted, my goal had been to hurry up and gain weight so I could get the hell out of there. But now I had a healthier motivation: to discover this whole new world outside the little box I'd grown up in.

October 6, 1991

(By now I had been given a discharge date of October 12.)

Talked with Alex today. It looks like I'll be going to Wyoming the first week of December. While we were on the phone, he said "dammit" to his dog, and it made me think of my father. He used to say "God dammit" all the time when he got mad. I'm not positive, but I think Alex's voice even resembles my father's.

After I got out of the hospital, I slowly settled back into some semblance of a normal life. My new routine included "aftercare" and Overeaters Anonymous meetings (there were no support groups specifically for anorexics). My new routine included "aftercare" and Overeaters Anonymous meetings (there were no support groups specifically for anorexics), to make sure I didn't slip back into my bad habits. I wasn't able to return to my radio station job right away, because my boss didn't trust that I was healthy (or mentally stable) enough yet. So, I had plenty of time on my hands. Besides planning my big trip out west, I also tried to locate Dad before meeting his family. I hoped to bring them good news about my father.

October 28, 1991

Yesterday Mom made reservations at a Boston hotel for next month. I can't tell you how many times she has made reservations and then cancelled them at the last minute, because she just decided not to go. She's never been to Boston. It's a very historic city. Plus, <u>everyone</u> in music is from there: Aerosmith, Bell Biv Devoe, Bobby Brown, Marky Mark, Extreme, etc. Of course, the number one reason for going is to find my father. Mom keeps saying he won't be there anymore, but maybe somebody knows where he went. Maybe the Boston Police can help.

I found a card in my grandmother's attic that my father sent me for my twelfth birthday. Inside, he wrote a message about remembering that I am American first, by birth, and that just about everyone here is of mixed heritage. I remember my mother and I being baffled by this at the time. Now, I think it's kind of spooky. Here I am with this complex of not knowing if I'm half-Mexican, or Spanish or what, and how it affected me growing up. Maybe my dad has trouble accepting his nationality, too. I need to find him so bad! He always promised to answer whatever questions I had when I was "old enough to understand." I'm pretty sure I still have that in writing someplace. Maybe he just needs to be reminded.

The stress of the upcoming trips, missing the friends I'd made in the hospital, and not having a job to go back to caused me to relapse into my disordered eating patterns within a month of my release. I was bingeing and purging and feeling depressed. I felt like my whole life's meaning rested on whether or not we made it to Boston. My journal entries during this time were full of suicidal ramblings.

My mother did not back out at the last minute this time. I reminded her that she'd promised in family counseling that she would stand by me.

"I'll take you, but *I* don't want to see him," she finally consented.

Somehow, Mom was able to find out that that Dad's last address had been some sort of halfway house. I was shocked. Mom, not so much. I had heard horror stories about such shelters in New York City, how many of the homeless felt safer sleeping on the streets, because they'd end up getting robbed in those places. Was Boston just as bad? I worried about my Dad being the victim of a violent crime or freezing to death in the winter. Phone calls to the shelter were fruitless; whoever answered the phone was protective of the privacy of the residents there. They wouldn't divulge any information. I was hung up on many times.

Mom and I only stayed in Boston for a day or two. We easily found the address in Brookline where Dad had last been known to reside, but as we suspected, he was no longer there. A woman who worked there told us it used to be a rooming house. More recently, it had been converted into a "guest house," although I couldn't tell you the difference. She gave us the phone number of the manager, who might be able to look up the records. I wrote in my journal that day:

November 9, 1991

We came home today. The trip was a drag. We didn't find Bob. We found the address with no problem. At the time my father lived there, it was a rooming house. Now it's a guest house.

I wanted to go to different stores and show his picture to different employees, to see if they remember him, but Mom wouldn't let me. I was rather angry with her. I'd also like to talk to the Brookline police. Could he qualify as a missing person? I doubt it. I wonder if he still lives in Massachusetts. Could he even be in New York somewhere? Maybe he's secretly watching me. I wonder what I'll say when I find him. What will he say? He can't turn me away. I won't let him.

I wasn't the only one chasing false leads. The family out west were going through the same ordeal.

November 20, 1991

Another one of my uncles, Anthony, says he may have located Bob! And in Florida, yet! Please let it be true. Please let him want to see me. Shit, I don't think I'd even recognize him if he passed me on the street. I wonder how much he's changed.

Florida, like so many hopeful possibilities before, turned out to be a dead end.

All that was left to do was move forward. That meant packing my bags for Wyoming. I was plenty nervous, not only about meeting all these strangers, but also because I had a phobia of flying. Being quite the pessimist at the time, I was sure the plane would crash, and that I'd die without meeting my relatives OR finding my father.

The morning of my flight, I wrote about feeling physically ill with anxiety:

December 6, 1991

I feel like I'm going to puke all over myself. I slept maybe one hour last night. I called a friend at work last night, just to talk, and he told me to just think of all the planes that land safely every day.

I even went on to say that I'd written out my will the night before! Needless to say, my worst nightmare did not come true. Hours later, my plane took off from La Guardia airport. By the time we reached our stop-over city, Atlanta, I was marveling at how pretty the city looked from up in the sky.

Next stop: Salt Lake City, Utah.

Chapter 6

Wyoming

I never knew much about my father's family at all, including my heritage. Was I Mexican? Was I Spanish? I was never given a direct answer. My Grandpa Newalis was a very prejudiced man. African-Americans were referred to as the N-word. He talked about "lazy Mexicans" and thought women were inferior to men. My mother kept the fact that my father was of Hispanic heritage secret from him... and from me. I had inherited Dad's dark skin and jet-black hair. There was no question that I was *something*. Mom lied and told Grandpa and me that I was Italian, and we both believed her. Still, I took a lot of cruel teasing in grade school, because I looked different. Looking at my first and second grade class photos, I was the only non-white child in my class. How I wished I were fair-skinned like my mom! When I was in junior high, a boy in one of my classes made a remark I'll never forget: "Holly used to be white, but she just doesn't take baths."

Mom must have inherited some of Grandpa's biases to a degree. One of her big worries was that here I was, fresh out of the eating disorders unit, and the Cordova clan would force me to eat Mexican food. The anxiety rubbed off on me. I worried that Grandma Cordova might make me eat burritos and other fattening things. Later, I finally learned that my family was Spanish. (I was told that I might even have some Apache in me, but no one in the family had ever been able to prove it.)

I flew into Salt Lake City, where I also had lots of relatives. Ironically, Salt Lake City is known for its largely Mormon population, and most of them are Jehovah's Witnesses! I was too busy meeting everyone and visiting their homes and sightseeing to do much journaling on this trip

Finding My Father

December 7, 1991

What an experience this is! I am staying at my Uncle Anthony's house. So far I have met Trina, Anthony (of course), Gerald, Lydia and Elaine, plus some of the kids: Mario, Reyna, and Jesse. Elaine is my favorite so far.

December 8, 1991

Today I met Aunt Rose and Uncle Paul, and about two dozen other relatives. I can't believe they all fit into that tiny home! Today we head to Rock Springs, Wyoming. No time to write now.

Later that day, met my paternal grandparents. By that time, everything was so surreal, I felt as though I were having an out-of-body experience. I had to keep pinching myself.

Wow... Here I am at my Grandma and Grandpa's house. What a weird feeling. Almost like déjà vu. I'm so comfortable here, it's like I've been here before. They're so nice! Especially Grandma. They don't look as old as they are. I also met Uncle Alex tonight. He smelled like my father: like beer. Boy, you should have seen the family guzzling the booze last night! It must run in the family.

Right now, there is a picture of my father staring at me from across the room, as I lay here on the couch. It's from when he was really young and in the Army. It doesn't even look like the Bob I remember.

The following day was spent with even more newly discovered relatives, doing Christmas shopping at the Cottonwood Mall in Salt Lake City. The family doted on me so much, they insisted on paying for some of my purchases, much to my surprise and delight. They wrestled me into one of those "Glamour Shots" type places, where they do your makeup and hair and take a photo shoot, airbrushing it to make you look like a movie star. I never did see the final product, although the relatives promised they'd mail copies of the pictures to me.

I also found out where I got my knack for songwriting. I have always been a creative and expressive person, and it frustrated me that my mother didn't seem to understand my poetry or my dark, moody song lyrics. She had no talent for art at all, and could never find the right words to express herself. She always used to say: "I don't know where you get it from." Apparently, I got it from Dad's side of the family. The family was full of musicians, including Gerald, who was in several local bands, and my cousins Elaine and Valerie, who both played guitar and sang. Elaine and Valerie were the daughters of my father's oldest brother, Henry, the only sibling that was deceased.

December 9, 1991

Elaine is the coolest person I've met here. She's so vibrant and vivacious. She talks up a storm and sings and plays the guitar. At the get-together at Rose's last night, she practically forced me to do two of my songs for the family. They enjoyed it, but it was sooo embarrassing!! Elaine has two girls. The little one is hearing-impaired. She's so sweet. She kept giving me her kitty cat to hold.

There were so many children in the family! They all wanted to meet me, play with me, and give me things. On Mom's side of the family, I only have two cousins, Jesse and Zac, my Uncle Bill's boys. I'd only met them two or three times in my life. We never really "clicked" as kids and didn't stay in touch. What a difference between that side of the family and my Dad's! Suddenly, I was surrounded by a bevy of adorable children, who thought the world of me.

The relatives showed me some old photographs… with me in them. They were taken the one other time they'd met me. I was a baby, and my parents had been driving from Seattle to settle back in New York. They made a family pit stop along the way.

Finding My Father

December 11, 1991

Today I got to meet my Aunt Jeannie, who I've see holding me in some of my baby pictures. She and my mother used to be good friends. She has four boys: Eddie, David, Daniel and Joey.

My Aunt Chevela and Uncle Lenny came over to the house last night with their two girls, Cierra and Jessica. Cierra is a three-year-old Shirley Temple look-alike. Jessica is about fourteen. She was full of questions about what New York City was like.

Uncle Alex is picking me up later today, to take me to see Jackson Hole, Wyoming. It's a three-hour drive. Sounds boring to me, but supposedly, I'll love the mountains and the elk. Yippee.

My whole Wyoming/ Utah experience was completely the opposite of how I grew up. There were never any reunions or get-togethers. I'm obviously an only child. My mom's brother and his family lives in Minnesota and hardly ever visited us on Long Island because of Grandpa Newalis. While my maternal grandfather had lots of brothers and sisters, he was always on the outs with them. As for Grandma Newalis, her sister, Katherine, had died of lung cancer before I was even born. She had a couple of cousins, but they weren't close with one another. So, excluding the short time Mom was married to Bud, the only family I ever had consisted of four people: Grandma, Grandpa, Mom and me. Unlike the Cordovas, there were never hugs and kisses or even much conversation. Everyone seemed to have a wall around them. We co-existed in our own little worlds, under one roof.

As I boarded the plane that would carry me home, I kept hearing my newfound grandmother's words in my head. Over and over again, she said: "I want to see Junior one more time, before I die." She was very emotional about it. Her husband was a little more reserved on the topic. I got the impression that while he respected his wife's wishes, he harbored some anger at my father for deserting the family. Rightfully so.

Sadly, I was not able to help make my grandmother's dream came true. Grandpa Cordova passed away in 1994, and Grandma Cordova died in 2001, long before I found my father. I fell out of touch with the Cordova family over the years, but that is changing, thanks to my dad.

Chapter 7

Chasing Shadows

Author's note: Some names in this chapter have been changed to protect the privacy of individuals involved.

Back home with Mom, I redoubled my efforts to find Dad, fueled by not only my needs, but by the expectations of his family. Meanwhile, there was plenty of drama on Mom's side of the family.

My Grandpa Newalis took a fall down the basement stairs in 1994. From then on, he was in a nursing home until his death later that year. My grandmother had been totally dependent on him. She couldn't drive a car. She did not know to write out a check. My mother and I temporarily moved back in with her, while we got rid of the decades of "stuff" that my grandfather had accumulated. He'd never allow us to buy anything new, from carpeting to modern appliances, nor did he ever throw anything out. He was a nightmare to buy for at Christmas, because he never wanted to use anything we gave him. Brand new shirts, ties and socks he'd received as gifts remained sealed in their packages and were stored in two dressers in his bedroom. Between those things, his tons of tools, and the household furniture, we had one hell of a yard sale!

Mom was excited that for the first time in her life, she would have enough money to purchase her own home. Up 'til then, life had always been a struggle for us financially, moving from one rented house or apartment to another. Mom purchased a nice ranch home in Southold. It wasn't far from Mattituck, but I worried that this would make it even less likely that I'd ever reconnect with Dad. All of his correspondence had come to me via my grandparents' P.O. Box in Mattituck. If he still had my address at all, it would be that one. Mom tried to reassure me that anything Dad sent would be forwarded to our new address. I hoped so.

Here is a journal entry from November 11, 1994. I was seeing a therapist named Liz, who was helping me to cope with my depression and anxiety.

Another thing we discussed was my father, and if I wanted to find him or not. That's always in the back of my mind. She wanted to know what I remembered about him, if I knew where he could be now, when I last saw him, if I looked like him, etc. She asked if I miss him. I pondered that and decided that it's more of a curiosity. I really want to know why he cut off his whole family. At least I know it's not just me he's avoiding. Why <u>everybody</u>?!? Doesn't he ever miss his mother or his brothers and sisters? Did something happen to him? Did he go crazy? Iis he in jail? Does he have amnesia? The most important thing is: Do I have any half-siblings out there? God, I'd love them to death! Someone can't be a loner and a drifter all their life. My father must have settled down by now. I really must stop procrastinating and make an effort to find him, even if it costs money to track him down. First, I'll try finding him through the child support agency. That would be free. Gives me chills to think about doing something so important.

Grandma lived with Mom and me for the next three years, and all the while she was deteriorating mentally. I don't think she had Alzheimer's, but she got real phobic towards the end, not wanting to leave the house or handle any new gadget, such as the TV remote. It might have been some form of dementia. Ultimately, it was a series of strokes and a bad heart that took her life in 1997.

That same year, I continued my efforts to contact my father. On August 27, 1997, I wrote the following journal entry:

Mailed off a letter to Dear Ol' Dad this morning. On the return address, I wrote my PO Box number, town and zip code, but not my name. Happily, it wasn't required on the form where he signs for it. If he knows it's from me, he might not want it.

The letter came back stamped "Return to Sender." I still have it.

By now I was back working regularly at WLNG, an oldies station in Sag Harbor. I started out interning there straight out of high school and eventually I got a regular airshift. I didn't have access to a computer at work or at home, so I enlisted the help of a co-worker who did.

August 1, 1997

I left Frank a note in his mailbox, asking if he knew of any good missing person websites, with information on how to track someone down. When I came into work yesterday, he approached me with a stack of papers he'd printed out, speaking in hushed tones, like a spy. He gave me all the pages from this one site, which listed several options (such as drivers license, social security number, etc.) to use as a starting point. It also listed books on finding missing persons, birth parents, heirs, etc. Frank also handed me a phone number for a search service, which has a set fee of $69. Kinda steep... but then again, NOT, considering. I wonder if any part of that is refundable, if they can't find the party in question.

The most promising thing on the list was "marriage records." It said that in some states, this type of search would give you the birth date and social security number of both parties. It can be retrieved at the county courthouse of the city where the couple was wed. In my parents' case, Seattle. I talked Mom into calling Seattle information, to track down these records. A while later, Mom informed me that she'd been given the runaround, and had to call about six different places. Finally getting the right one, she had to deal with a "nasty" lady with a bad attitude. She huffily told Mom that they could not disclose any birth date or social security number to ANYONE. We CAN, however, obtain a copy of the marriage certificate by sending a written request. Might as well. Although, I advised Mom to rummage through her hope chest before we do this, because she MUST have it somewhere!

Another way you can track someone down is to use their traffic tickets to track down their current drivers license number. He got a lot of tickets. He often drove with a beer between his legs, I recall. He used to pull stunts like making U-turns in the middle of the road.

Would the County Center in Riverhead still have records going back to the '70s??

Hey! I just thought of something! He remarried after he moved to Boston. Maybe their marriage record would be easier to track down than the Seattle one!

Later that month...

August 25, 1997

Big news. I think I found my father! Frank got something off the computer for me, after my search panned out to nothing. This search was more expansive than the first. The service's phone number had a 718 area code. I thought it was in Boston, but Mom said no, it's upstate New York.

When I dialed it, initially I spoke with a woman who can an indiscernible accent. She kept asking me to spell everything over and over. Then a man (her supervisor, I presume) got on the phone and repeated what she'd written down, to see if it was correct. It wasn't. She'd written "Adelphi" instead of Adolph, for one thing. Armed with accurate spellings, the man said goodbye and he'd be in touch soon. An hour later, he called back and said: "We've found him."

I was reeling! This was impossible! After dozens of family members had tried to track him down for years, I've found him in a matter of hours?!? This is too good to be true. I'm so scared to get me hopes up.

According to the man, whose name was Robert, I think, my father is still living in Massachusetts. Then, to my complete shock and utter bafflement, Robert revealed that they'd also found an address for him in Hawaii. HAWAII?!? That's the most expensive place in the U.S.A. to live! My father could never even keep a job! The jobs he did get were menial labor, like washing dishes in local restaurants. Robert declared that this Hawaii address was active as recently as last year! What did he do; win the lottery?!?

Robert says that my father is 56 years old. There is no mention of a new wife or any other children. They'll be faxing some stuff to my workplace that I'll have to sign. I will have to contact my father via certified letter. Robert asked me if it was okay to let my dad know that I was looking for him. I wasn't sure how to answer that. My fear of being rejected is huge. So, what am I to do? Take another trip to Boston and just show up on his doorstep? I guess a letter is my best bet. I just hope he'll at least open it and read it before throwing it away or sending it back, marked: "Return to Sender." I don't mean to sound so pessimistic, but I have learned that when it comes to getting happy or excited about anything, "Not So Fast" is the best motto.

"Not so fast" was right. It turned out to be a dead address. I cannot find the journal I kept from that period of my life, but suffice to say I was devastated. (By the way, my dad never lived in Hawaii. Maybe he and his second wife honeymooned there? I have no clue where that bit of info came from!)

My twenties were an emotional roller-coaster ride. Mom and I continued to live together, as I didn't make enough money working at the radio station to move out on my own. She and I were often at odds with each other. A lot of it was my fault. I have suffered from depression since I was an adolescent. This manifested itself in many ways. There was the on-again-off-again eating disorder, Body Dysmorphic Disorder, suicidal thoughts, anti-social tendencies and burning/ cutting. Thank God I had my writing for an outlet, or I guarantee you I would be dead right now. I filled notebook after notebook, journal after journal with documentation of my misery. Also, there was music. I'd sometimes write as many as ten songs a day, mostly very dark, brooding, negative stuff. It was therapy of sorts, but I could never shake the sadness completely. I was sure I'd inherited whatever mental illness my father might have had.

I continued to see therapists throughout the 1990s for my eating disorders. I was in group therapy with a counselor named Eve for a period in the late 90s. There were maybe half a dozen other women, from all walks of life, who participated in these sessions. We talked about family issues, our feelings about ourselves and our struggles with food and body image. Even though we all had different backgrounds, careers, and lifestyles, we were bound by our abnormal food and body image issues. And there was another things we had in common. After a particularly emotional session, where all of us shared painful memories from our childhood, one of the women, Erin, made the remark: "None of us came from good fathers. Isn't that sad?"

Here's an excerpt from a journal entry I made on February 2, 1999, two days after my 27th birthday.

Mom's theory is that Dad has remarried, perhaps to a woman with "a little money." I don't believe THAT for a second. Why would a rich woman even go out with, let alone marry, a reclusive alcoholic who can't even hold on to a minimum wage job? Nothing makes sense. I sent off a postcard the other day. Wonder if you can stamp a postcard "Return To Sender"? I hope not! How will I know if he got it/ is still there, etc.?

Something missing from my story so far, you might have noticed, is the absence of any boyfriends. I'd only been with one boy before, when I was 17. Both of us had simply wanted to lose our virginity, so we used each other. I'd never had any relationships after that until I was in my early twenties. Once I did start pursuing some intimate relationships (here's where we get into some deep Freudian territory), I dated guys that were, if not old enough to be my father, damn close to it. And, for the most part, they shared my dad's more unsavory traits.

First, there was Joe, who I knew from work. Twelve years my senior, Joe was a gigolo who could not be faithful to any one woman. He was also an alcoholic, who, try as he may, could not stay sober for long. He was always on the run from people he owed money to. Even though I wasn't earning enough to live on my own, I would "loan" him $75 at the drop of a hat. (I use quotation marks here, because I knew perfectly well that he'd never pay me back.) If I didn't say yes and give him the money he needed, I'd probably never see him. If it meant that I'd get to see Joe, even if were just for a few, fleeting moments at the bus stop in Southampton, I'd give him anything he wanted. If I was lucky, we'd get to sit down and have a coffee together at a little corner café called The Golden Pear. But Joe was always nervously looking around, worrying about who was there to see us. I was never permitted to visit him at the house where he rented a room, supposedly because his landlord was a crazy old man who was a compulsive hoarder. "There are stacks of old newspapers up to the ceiling. He doesn't let anyone in there," he explained. Joe had a bad habit of disappearing for a week, or more, seemingly dropping off the face of the earth. During these times, I would agonize as to his possible whereabouts, imagining that he might be dead of an overdose, or beaten and left to die by one of his enemies. Usually, though, he'd just relapsed. Eventually, he'd call me, usually from rehab. I had to just let him go.

2/24/99

Depressed. I feel loss and lost, rejected and neglected. Emotionally ravenous for paternal love, and a thirst for family that will never be quenched. It's hard, when I am doing everything in my power and still coming up empty-handed.

Every day, when Mom goes to the post office, I'd be happy when stuff came, and disappointed if I didn't get anything. I'd celebrate the arrival of materials relating to my songwriting. But I was really blocking out the reality of no news from my father.

My father has not responded or acknowledged me. Why did I think this time would be any different? My feeling is this: if I can't get my own father to give me the time of day, how can I expect any man to love or respect me? Mom says it has nothing to do with that, but it's got EVERYTHING to do with it! A girl's relationship with her father shapes all her future relationships with men. If he coddles and pampers her, she expects it from every man... like a Sugar Daddy. If he's abusive, she'll find a guy who beats her.

For poor as-good-as-orphans like me, who had no, or hardly any father at all, she'll always be seeking that father figure who isn't there, whether it's an actual much-older man, or someone who's controlling and domineering. Whatever image she's created in her head of what a "father" is. And, of course, none of them is ever good enough.

With Joe, the whole sh-bang was there: the drinking, the disappearing act, the childlike dependency, etc. I was under the impression Bob only drank beer. But Mom says: "Sometimes he drank the hard stuff, too."

I went on to express my desire to hire a lawyer, who perhaps could *force* my father to speak to me, even if it was through a middleman. There was medical information I felt I was entitled to. I wanted to know if my NF (Neurofibromatosis) had been inherited from him. I was even more worried that I might be genetically prone to whatever mental health issues afflicted my father. I had already pretty much decided by that time that I didn't want children, but in case I changed my mind, I wanted to know if there were any disorders or diseases that ran in our family.

My next romantic conquest was Rob, a musician and studio engineer. He and I worked on lots of music together. He was maybe seventeen years older than me. I'd gone to school with two of his nieces (Ironically, one of them had NF). Rob could be accurately described as a "tortured genius." He fought a courageous battle with depression. He tried to stay on top of it with all-natural and holistic medicines. He kept a basket of vitamins and St. John's Wort in his kitchen, part of his half-hearted attempt to get well. We shared a common bond there, albeit a dangerous one. One time, he almost broke my heart when he told me: "We're spiraling each other down." Like Joe before him, Rob was an alcoholic. He managed to stay sober most of the time. The only time I saw him relapse was when I came to a recording session and found him in the basement, staring at a pyramid of empty beer cans.

Incongruously, Rob was a Reiki Master. Reiki is a form of therapy which means "universal life energy" in Japanese. He could heal people (and even animals, he told me) of physical and spiritual pain or distress by laying his hands directly on, or hovering over, certain body parts. Of course, I wanted him to lay his hands on me, but Rob wouldn't do this unless I agreed to go to one of his Reiki meetings with him. I declined. Too mysta-magical, metaphysical, hocus-pocus-y for my tastes. Besides, I'd seen a picture of Regina, the woman who led the meetings with him. With her dark hair and tan complexion, she bore a striking resemblance to Rob's ex-wife, Shelley. Rob never got over his ex. The divorce destroyed him. I'd seen photographs of Rob and Shelley when they were married. She had olive skin and black hair, like Regina. And like me. I wondered if Rob was just gravitating towards women who looked like his former wife. I was extremely jealous of both Shelley and Regina.

When not making music together, Rob and I would talk and laugh and discuss everything under the sun: current events, work, family, our childhoods, movies and sex. My relationship with Rob remained a platonic one, although I tried diligently to make him love me as a woman, and not just a friend. He touched, he teased, he cuddled, he drove me crazy with desire, but he never would go as far as I wanted him to. In the end, he wound up committing suicide.

My next love interest, Sam, was older yet, by about twenty years. (Was I subconsciously thinking of how my father was growing older? Would this explain the noticeable upward progression in the age of my boyfriends?) At least Sam had no substance abuse or mental health issues. He was my first "nice" boyfriend. He treated me with utmost respect and I guess I boosted his self-esteem, him being in his mid-forties and me being a young twenty-something with the hots for him! We went out to dinner quite often. This helped me immensely, as far as my food issues were concerned. I learned how to connect food with love and fun, and not calories and fat grams.

This relationship had promising beginnings, but things started to fall apart after a year. Sam was a workaholic, for one thing. And, eventually, he could not get past the age difference. He once told me I made him feel like a "dirty old man!" I never did figure out if he was joking or not. Even more troubling, he didn't want to introduce me to his teenage daughter. She was his pride and joy. He was constantly bragging about her academic accomplishments. I was jealous. Not of Sam's daughter, but of this demonstration of a father's love that I had lacked all my life. Our relationship fizzled out in a natural sort of way. We just started seeing less and less of each other, until we stopped trying to make our schedules match. We still emailed and talked on the phone often, long after we had ceased being "secret lovers." It was the first of any of my relationships where we remained friends after breaking up.

Chapter 8

Finding Myself

Around this period, I found myself feeling stagnated; trapped in the past and sinking in the present. I rented a couple of rooms in Sag Harbor, first with an eccentric British woman who was a movie director; then with an elderly lady who was a huge Patsy Cline fan. After a few months, I was back living with Mom in Hampton Bays, unable to afford rent and living expenses on my paltry salary.

Money issues aside, I was at the end of my rope at work. I couldn't get a raise. I didn't feel valued or respected as a woman. I knew that the antiquated equipment in the studio was a hindrance to my future in radio. Everything there was ancient; nothing digital, no computers. We were still using "cart machines" (each song, jingle and commercial was on what looks like an 8-track tape) and reel-to-reel tapes. It was a huge deal when we got two CD players in the studio. I never thought I'd live to see the day! I didn't want to be unable to get a job at another station in the future because of my lack of knowledge of modern technology.

On top of that, I had a nasty co-worker at the station that was obsessed with me and had been stalking and harassing me. He eventually got fired, but the emotional toll it had taken on me was enormous. I was seeing yet another therapist to deal with the stressful situation, but even she never knew how ravaged I was by the whole mess. I was suicidal during this period. Even after the employee got fired, I didn't feel victorious. I felt as though I'd been emotionally raped.

I tried applying at another radio station in the Hamptons and actually got offered a job, but not for very much more money. My WLNG boss talked me into staying, with a wee bit of a raise. But I had to stop kidding myself. There still was no way I could afford to live in the Hamptons, or even on the more rural North Fork.

What reasons did I have to continue living on Long Island? Rob was dead, Sam and I had drifted apart, and Mom and I were driving each other crazy, living under the same roof. The job situation sucked, even with Stalker Dude out of the picture. I needed to grow and flourish, and I felt like I was wilting instead.

Knowing I had to take action or be left in the dust, I signed up for computer classes. I knew that I'd need computer skills if I wanted to get hired anywhere, regardless of what kind of job I ended up doing. I was an eager student and fast learner, mostly because I felt like I needed to do it to save my life, or rather, to start a new one.

My next step was to start looking for radio job listings I online. I sent my resume and demo CD of my air shift to maybe half a dozen stations, at most. By then, I'd completely switched musical tastes from oldies and alternative rock to contemporary country. I was hell-bent on getting a job at a country station. A few months after I'd sent my package out, I received a phone call from a country station in upstate NY… 400 miles from home.

I moved up to Watertown, NY in August of 2001. I'd done extensive research on the area and was awestruck by the difference in the cost of living. I could finally afford to be independent! I made two trips upstate before making my decision; once with Sam and then with Mom.

I rented a nice apartment within walking distance of my new workplace. Everything was so different than on Long Island! I had to get used to the new job, the names of strange towns, the North Country accents, the much more laid-back lifestyle… it was a whole new world. I settled into it comfortably. I found a writers' group to join. I sang in a band, Neon Connection for a short time (we even got to open for country star Aaron Tippin once!). And. Most importantly, I was living out my dream of working at a country station, doing the mid-day shift at Froggy 97. We all had "Froggy" names that we used on the air, such as James Pond, Webb Foote and Jumpin' Jay. Mine was "Cricket." It suited me, because I'm so small!

My first boyfriend up north was another poor choice. Johnny was a part-timer at the radio station, a redneck rebel without a cause, originally from North Carolina. His southern accent, badass attitude and the fact that he was a guitar player all appealed to me. Johnny's childhood had been even more unstable than mine. He grew up bouncing in and out of children's homes, occasionally living with relatives, and sometimes fending for himself out on the streets. We gravitated towards each other, whether it was because of our sordid pasts, or because we were both newcomers in an unfamiliar city, or maybe just because there was a sexual chemistry between us that couldn't be ignored. I remember the first time I met him, hearing his unique laugh and observing his rebellious, mischievous personality, thinking, "I am going to sleep with this guy." Never mind the fact that he was married. He and his wife were separated; I am many things, but I'm NOT a homewrecker! Before I knew it, Johnny had moved into my apartment. This was the first time I lived with a guy, and my first long-term relationship with a guy my own age.

There were problems from the get-go. Johnny hated authority. He loved beer, pot and for a short time, me. I loved him too. But his temper, coupled with my immaturity and impatience was a bad combination. We lasted a few months, before Johnny got fed up and left me. I was devastated. I begged him, groveled to him not to go.

"You'll be just *fiiine*," he assured me in his thick southern drawl, before disappearing into the night forever.

I wrote a song called "Wasted Time" about the breakup. In the chorus, I compared Johnny to my father:

Tell me that it all meant something
Say it wasn't all for nothing
Tell me why you had to leave
Like my deadbeat dad abandoned me...

I wrote that song in 2002. When I demoed it, I wouldn't let the background vocalist sing with me on that last line; I felt I had to sing it alone, because it was so personal. Years later. I'd find out it was also misinformed.

I'm convinced that there's no way I could have chosen healthy relationships from the get-go, given my lack of positive male role models growing up. From an alcoholic, absentee father, to a strict, intimidating stepfather (who also drank too much), to a controlling, emotionally abusive grandfather who overstepped his boundaries in ways I can't even bring myself to mention. I knew nothing else of men. "Good Dads" were fictional characters on TV sitcoms. Romantic, attentive lovers were the fodder of cheesy soap operas. In the real world, men were not to be trusted to be faithful or to stick around.

I had a new computer at the time (a case of me and Johnny living above our means. And who do you think got stuck with the payments?), and it proved to be a valuable tool in finding two very important men in my life: my father and my future husband.

As more and more information about everything and everybody became available online, I found many search services that promised to "find almost anyone." Since they were all new and novel at the time, they offered special low fees. I chose one I'd heard at work, advertised on our radio station. In 2001, I hit pay dirt. The last address listed for my father was in Dorchester, Massachusetts!

I was able to find out that the place that he was staying was an assisted living facility for seniors. This struck me as odd, as he wasn't that old (mid-60s) at the time. I wrote to my father, basically just telling him where I lived now and what I did for a living. I wasn't sure if he'd write back or not. After all I'd been through, I expected it to be another false lead. But lo and behold, this time he wrote back! He was happy to hear from me and relieved that I was doing alright. He even asked how Mom was doing. My father had never really abandoned me after all. We'd just sort of lost each other. But I still had to piece together how everything could have fallen apart to the extent it did.

Dad's notes were never long. He rarely wrote more than a few sentences in the cards that he sent. He didn't really acknowledge the span of time that had gone by. It's like we picked up right where we'd left off after taking a lunch break in a game of Monopoly. It was somewhat bizarre. Then again, little of anything to do with my father had ever made much sense. I just rolled with the flow.

Dad sent me some photographs of himself. One was a wedding picture of him and his second wife, Pamela. He still looked young in the photo. I guessed that it had been taken in the late 1980s. He wrote on the back of the picture that Pamela had died. Epilepsy or Cerebral Palsy, I can't remember which. There were two other photos of Dad standing outside. In one, he was alone. In another, he was posing with a friend of his, who was dressed as Santa Claus. I looked closely at my father's face. He'd aged well. He might be down and out, but he still had a dapper appeal to him. He looked a lot like Grandpa Cordova, actually. He wanted me to keep the pictures, but I had copies made and sent them back to him. I didn't want to take away the only mementos that he had.

Eventually, I got to speak with him on the phone, after making arrangements with his caseworker. "Nervous" and "butterflies" do not even scrape the surface of the anxiety I had about actually speaking with him on the phone. I would have been less nervous giving an oral presentation in front of a million people! I couldn't rationalize my fear, especially after the long, frustrating chase over tens of years and hundreds of miles. Surprisingly, he didn't want to stay on the phone too long. Like the notes he sent me in the mail, he kept his conversations brief. He told me that he'd been worried about me all those years we were apart, and wanted to know how I was doing, and how Mom was doing.

But when I told Dad I did radio for a living, he said something very strange: "Oh, I *thought* that was your voice I heard in the bar!" he remarked. I didn't even know what to say. I knew that something was very wrong. My father's claim was impossible. Froggy's signal didn't reach Boston. At that time, we weren't even streaming online. Besides, Dad hadn't heard me speak since I was a little girl. How could he have recognized my voice?

I would come to learn that Dad hears a lots of "voices."

After that awkward conversation, I hardly ever answered the phone when I saw the 617 area code on my caller ID. It was avoidance, and not the right thing to do, but I didn't know how else to deal with my father's unreality. I preferred to communicate with him via snail mail. Whenever we talked on the phone, my father would make perfect sense throughout most of the conversation, then all of a sudden, he'd get "out there." Frankly, it scared me.

Getting back to the ever-growing power of the internet, I had signed up for a lot of online dating services after Johnny left. I communicated with several lonely guys, but I only ever met one of them face to face. That person was Pete.

Pete was eight years older than me, recently divorced, and the non-custodial father of an eleven-year-old girl. Having recently been laid off from his factory job, Pete was unemployed when we first started dating, except for his occasional music gigs (he's a bass player). This didn't bother me as much as the fact that he was *nice*. I wasn't used to a ready smile, good manners and thoughtfulness. Pete fell for me long before I fell for him. I resisted him and tested him and fought him every step of the way. He was the opposite of everything I'd ever known. He came from a "normal" family. His mom and dad had been married for more than forty years and still lived in the same house where he'd grown up. Everyone was close and involved in one another's lives (with the exception of Pete's weird brother, Rick, who does his own thing).

My mother was a big factor in encouraging me to let Pete into my heart. She spoke with Pete a few times on the phone before they met in person. Mom sold her house in Hampton Bays and moved up to Watertown in 2003. Like me, she had gotten sick of the high cost of living on Long Island and joined me up north. She got into the landlord business, supporting herself by renting out apartments in the three multi-family houses that she purchased. She and I lived in a side-by-side duplex on a nice, quiet street. Living apart for a couple of years had actually brought Mom and I closer. She had made peace with the past and was all about living in the moment now. She'd retired from her work as a home heath aide, so she was free to pursue her hobbies… namely, hitting all of the area casinos! For the first time in our lives, my mother and I were truly friends.

Mom liked Pete right away. She embarrassed me during our very first outing together. We were all in the car and had stopped at a convenience store. I ran inside to get a coffee. Pete later told me that while I was in the store, my mother turned to him and blurted out: "So, are you going to ask Holly to marry you?"

Chapter 9

Man and Wife

Pete and I were wed on May 22, 2004. For lack of a father, my mother gave me away. I don't regret this, because she never looked more beautiful than she did on that day, in her royal blue pantsuit, perfectly coiffed hair and manicured nails. After Pete and I exchanged our wedding vows, Mom joined me and the other girls in my wedding party cutting up the dance floor to Gretchen Wilson's "Redneck Woman." The "old" Mom I had grown up with never would have done such a thing! She had always been so prim and reserved. In the last couple of years, Mom had loosened up so much, it was having a whole new mother! I have no idea what made her change, but I embraced the person she had become. While Mom still didn't like to talk about the past, she no longer hated my father. She thought it would be good for me to find him.

Shortly after Pete and I started dating, he unexpectedly regained custody of Caitlin. He worried that this would cause a rift between he and I, since I'd specified in my online dating ad that I was looking for a man with no kids, or a non-custodial father. But everything worked out fine. At the time, Caitlin was a happy-go-lucky kid, and we got along fine. (This was before she hit her teens.) She was part of our wedding party, and looked very grown-up in her royal blue gown.

I now had in-laws, Pete and Barb. I liked them both. They were very active senior citizens who enjoyed camping and the outdoors. I had to get used to their "different" lifestyle, which was foreign to me, compared to the way I'd grown up. They had lots of animals (dogs, cats, fish, what have you), whereas I hadn't been allowed to have pets during my childhood (other than the ones we'd left with my stepfather). The Gaskins had holiday family traditions, whereas my family just went through the motions on such occasions. I liked to listen to Barb and Pete banter back and forth, exchanging little one-liners and zingers that amused me to no end. My parents and grandparents had never talked to each other that way. Instead, there was either awkward silence or arguments. I grew up in an environment that was pretty much devoid of a sense of humor. So time spent in the Gaskin family environment was a little bit of a welcome culture shock!

I called Barb by her first name, but I had a dilemma about what to call my father-in-law. I didn't want to call him "Pete," because it would be too confusing, since that's also my husband's name. "Pop" just isn't me, and "Pa" is what Mom called my grandfather. I couldn't bring myself to call him "Dad." I'd feel like I was betraying my real father by doing so. I write "Old Pete" on his Christmas gifts, but to this day, when I talk directly to my father-in-law, I don't call him anything at all.

In 2006, Pete and I started making plans to visit Boston to see my father. Everything was tentative, as it was hard to arrange time off from our jobs (me at the radio station and Pete at a car dealership). Finding someone to watch Caitlin was another challenge. The in-laws could be relied on to watch her for a day or two, but not for an extended period. Her own mother (Pete's ex) was not very reliable. Additionally, we were just about keeping our heads above water financially, between paying our bills and mortgage payments and Caitlin's needs. At one point, my mother shocked me by offering to take me there herself! I told her no, Pete and I would find a way to make the trip.

Then, the unthinkable happened. On December 12, 2006, my mother, Lillian Olmsted, was killed in a car accident. She was 64 years old. My mother had had her share of fender benders in her lifetime, but this was totally and devastatingly unexpected. It was such a freak thing, because she always worried about driving in the wintry North Country weather, yet this was a beautiful, sunny, snow-free day. She died on her brother's birthday, and one day before my mother-in-law's birthday. Needless to say, my whole world was turned upside down.

My boss insisted I take the rest of the year off. I needed it. Not so much emotionally, because I was in shock, operating on auto-pilot.

But Pete and I found that my mom's state of affairs was such a mess, it was almost too much for us to handle. She'd always been super-secretive about her finances, and with good reason, I found out. She owed tons of credit card debt.

Then there was all the "junk." My mother wasn't quite a "hoarder," like the horrifying cases you may have seen on TV, but she was most definitely an extreme packrat. Sifting through her things as I was cleaning out her apartment, I found boxes upon bags of "stuff." I'm defining "stuff" here as things that take up space, which are never looked at, are forgotten about, are of no use whatsoever, which, if I threw away, Mom never would have missed them. However, if she'd caught me trying to throw them away, she would've pitched one hell of a fit. There were enough bills (all paid, but she kept the paperwork) to start a small landfill. Dozens of cards, letters and used-up puzzle books. Souvenirs and trinkets from the casinos she loved to frequent. Pay stubs from the phone company where she'd worked in the 1960s. Legal papers and love letters. Christmas presents she'd never taken out of the boxes, and clothing with the tags still on. Certificates of merit from the various home health agencies she'd worked for in the '80s...

And tons of pictures.

Most of the photographs I recognized. There were lots of my old baby pictures and class photos. Others were black and white shots of relatives I never knew. Mom had pics from trips she'd taken without me, photos of old friends and pets, and of the developmentally disabled adults she'd worked with in one of her former careers. Most fascinating to me was a certain portrait taken sometime in 1971. Although she had told me that she and my father had never had a wedding photo taken, what to my wondering eyes should appear? You guessed it! I was shocked to discover the picture of Mom in a pretty lavender party dress and Dad in a suit and tie, posing for the camera with their wedding cake and a glass of wine! I wondered if Mom had kept it hidden from me on purpose all those years, or if she'd forgotten about it, packed away with the rest of her junk. He looked so handsome and she was beautiful, like a young Elizabeth Taylor.

I dragged myself through the soul-draining task of calling all of Mom's friends, distant relatives and her co-workers at the local nursing home, where she volunteered as a mail carrier. I think that was the hardest part of my mother's death; having to deliver such horrible news, and hearing the devastated reactions of those who loved her.

I had no idea how my father would react to the news. Would he even understand? I had spoken to him on the phone only a couple of times since moving to Watertown. He seemed so out of touch with reality that it upset me to speak with him. I preferred to write him letters, or deliver messages through his case worker. But news like this wasn't the kind of thing you break to someone over the phone or in a letter. This was Dad's former wife; the mother of his only child. I never got the impression, from Dad's letters over the years, that he harbored any ill feelings towards Mom. For all I knew, he might still love her a little.

Between agonizing over how to tell my Dad the sad news, Pete and I were overwhelmed with getting Mom's financial chaos in order. We'd also become instant landlords, trying to juggle and manage the three rental properties (all duplexes) we'd inherited when Mom died. We had to deal with nightmare tenants, some of whom trashed their apartments, and another who was sub-letting and dealing illegal drugs on our property. Then there was the shady handyman who'd already screwed my mother out of thousands of dollars, and who had the balls to call me up two days after she died, insisting that Mom had wanted to make him her property manager! It was just too much stress, and with all the repairs that constantly had to be done, Pete and I decided that the landlord business was not for us. One by one, we sold the houses off.

Meanwhile, Caitlin had grown into a difficult teenager. She bounced back and forth between our household and her mother's. She was constantly in trouble at school and her temper caused a lot of stress and friction in our home. This was another factor that made it difficult for us to travel. We had taken shorter trips in the past, only to have her break into the house when we weren't there and steal things.

Then there were my own health issues; my eating disorder had returned once again. I was hospitalized for nearly two weeks in early 2009.

It seemed like we'd never make it to Boston, but we did, two years later than originally planned.

Chapter 10

Reunited

Dad wrote to me sporadically. To his credit, he never, ever forgot my birthday on January 31st. However, the increasing illegibility of my father's handwriting worried both me and Pete. To say it was "messy" would be the understatement of the year. His penmanship had always been poor, but now it was what my mother would have called "chicken scratch." The letters were so shaky, I wondered if he had Parkinson's. His personal messages were getting shorter each time he wrote to me. Eventually, all he could write was "Your Dad, Adolph Cordova." Someone else addressed the envelope for him. I worriedly wrote back, asking him about his health, but he ignored my questions.

I spoke with his caseworker, a pleasant man named Leslie. The first time I called, he was surprised that I existed. "I didn't know Adolph had any family!" he exclaimed. That kind of hurt my feelings. Why wouldn't Dad have told his own case worker about me? I inquired as to my father's health. Leslie wasn't at liberty to divulge too much of my dad's personal information. "Adolph is very private," he said. One thing he did disclose, was that my father was in the early stages of Alzheimer's.

My heart sank into my stomach. In spite of the strange phone conversations I'd had with Dad since I tracked him down, I wasn't expecting news like this. I'd attributed his odd statements to what my mother had told me: "he'd just get 'out there' sometimes.'" But Alzheimer's? Suddenly, I was consumed with urgency. I knew only the basics about this disease, but it was clear to me that I couldn't afford to waste any more time.

Despite assurances from Dad's case manager, Leslie, that my father was excited to see me again, I was extremely nervous about visiting him. I wasn't sure how I felt about him. I wanted to believe that I loved him, but truthfully, he was a stranger. Add to that, the burden of being the bearer of bad news (my mother's death) and the fact that I'd never dealt with anyone who had Alzheimer's Disease before. I had no idea what to expect. I was so concerned that the trip might be a letdown, that I bought tickets to a concert (Keith Urban and Taylor Swift) at a Boston arena, and scheduled our trip around that. That way, even if my reunion with Dad didn't go well, there would still be something enjoyable about the trip. As it turned out, I needn't have worried.

The short story, Adolph, in the beginning of this book, is a dramatization. I wasn't actually alone during that scary taxi ride. My wonderful, supportive husband, Pete, was with me during that tense trip. I could not have done it by myself.

The heat was oppressive that day, yet there was Dad, in a long-sleeved dress shirt and a tie, waiting for us on a bench in front of his building. He looked as anxious as I felt. As much as he'd aged, I knew it was him right away. It was probably even easier for him to recognize me. I haven't changed that much since he last saw me; I still have the same long, straight, black hair and bangs that I had at five years old.

"Howdy," he said to me.

"Hi, Dad," I said. How long I'd waited to say that simple phrase!

We rushed into each other's arms, blinking back tears. Any doubt and awkwardness dissolved in that brief embrace. A lot of healing took place in that moment.

Telling my father about my mother's sad fate was nowhere near as difficult as I'd thought it would be. Inevitably, he asked me how she was. I meekly replied that she had passed away two years before. When I told him that she had been killed in a car accident, he exclaimed: "Oh, for Heaven's sake! She always *was* getting into car accidents." He shook his head in exasperation.

It was true; my mother had a history of fender benders. The worst one was well before I was born. She'd been hospitalized for two months as a result of a collision between her and a carload of teenagers, one of whom had died in the crash. She'd told me about it several times, specifically about how she never had a single visitor during the long, painful recovery period, not even her own parents. Grandpa assumed the crash must have been her fault. He punished her by not visiting her in the hospital, and didn't allow Grandma to go see her either. (As I mentioned, my grandmother didn't drive, although I imagine she must have been crazed with worry about her daughter.) Mom had to have a steel plate put in her right elbow, forcing her to give up one of her favorite hobbies, bowling. She had a horrific, Frankenstein-like scar that she was terribly self-conscious about. She also had an injury to her knee that gave her problems for the rest of her life.

On a brighter note, I was surprised to find out that a traffic mishap was how my mother and father had met! Dad told Pete and I the following delightful story over lunch.

"I was driving a taxi in Seattle, Washington, and this crazy madwoman crashed into the back end of my cab. Rather than have her arrested, I married her. I should have had her arrested!"

I'd forgotten how funny my dad was. When I was a little girl, he used to make me laugh until I wet my pants. With all he'd been through, his sense of humor was still in tact.

Dad, Pete and I were seated by the window in a restaurant called CF Donovan's. I couldn't remember the last time I'd eaten a meal with my father. Dad insisted on ordering the same thing I did, which was a grilled veggie wrap (I am a vegetarian). I felt bad, because I thought he would have much preferred a big, juicy hamburger.

I noticed that Dad had a very bad tremor on his right side. This explained the almost indecipherable handwriting in the cards and letters he'd sent me in recent years. It was constant. Dad regretted that the shaking prevented him from using a computer.

"I don't want you to think I'm computer illiterate," he said. "But it's so frustrating when I lose a whole program because I accidentally hit the wrong button."

The shaking was not due to Parkinson's, as I had feared.

"The doctors said it was a stroke," he explained, but he sounded skeptical. He told us that he didn't believe in doctors or medicine.

Great. Another thing to worry about. So my father was stubborn. Now I knew where I'd gotten it from!

The beginning stages of the Alzheimer's were evident. Many times in our conversation, my father would stop in the middle of a sentence and declare: "I forgot what I was going to say," or "I had so many questions I wanted to ask you, but I can't remember." He assured me that he'd think of it later, and usually he did. When walking through the neighborhood where he did his shopping, he explained how he would wrap a rubber band around his fingers to remind himself that he had errands to run. When he remembered to complete his errands, he'd take the rubber band off and put it back in his pocket.

My father asked the normal questions any loving dad would ask his long-long daughter. Did I finish high school? Did I have any children? Did I live in a good neighborhood? I explained to him about Caitlin (leaving out the details of her delinquency), and described our house, our jobs, our pets, and everything else.

One of his questions, which he asked me the second day of our visit, caught me off guard.

"Were you abused?" he asked.

I tried to hide my shock. I knew exactly what he was talking about.

My Grandpa Newalis, as I mentioned earlier, was brutally abusive to my mother and my uncle when they were kids. With me, the abuse was mostly psychological and verbal. "You'll never amount to anything," "you have no personality" and "you're gonna grow up to be fat and lazy like your mother" were typical statements. There were darker incidents of abuse as well, but I glossed over the truth for my father's benefit. I saw no need for him to know about the terrible things Grandpa said and did to me. Still, it killed me that he'd been worried about this for the past three decades. Of course, I also found myself falling into a pattern of useless "if only" thinking… *"If only my father had remained in my life, I wouldn't have had to go through all that."*

Some of my father's questions made it evident that he had difficulty processing time, in the sense of how many years had gone by. For instance, he asked me if my grandparents were still alive. They had been dead thirteen and sixteen years at that time. A "normal" person would have realized how unlikely it would be for them to still be living. Yet, he seemed more surprised that *they* were dead than when I told him my mom was! Likewise, he asked me if I knew if his own parents were living, and of course the answer was no, they had passed on. They had been even older than my maternal grandparents. Dad didn't show any noticeable emotion when I told him his folks were dead. He just said "oh."

I had questions that I wanted to ask him, but didn't, because it was too uncomfortable. Like, why did he cut his whole family out of his life? But what right did I have to ask him this, when I had done the same thing? After meeting them in 1992, I'd ceased communicating with them, except for when Aunt Virginia somehow tracked me down in the mid-1990s, to tell me of a death in the family. Nevertheless, I asked Dad if he wanted me to get in touch with his family for him. He hesitated a long time before answering. I held my breath.

"No," he said, decisively.

He went on to talk about his younger brother, Alex, and how he'd changed after being in Vietnam.

"He used to be so happy-go-lucky, such a nice, fun kid," he said. "But when he came back, he was never the same. He was stoic. You couldn't talk to him."

I didn't bother trying to reason with Dad that the trauma of war would do that to most anyone. I just agreed that when I had met Uncle Alex, yes, "stoic" was a good word to describe his personality.

I asked my father how come he didn't go by "Bob" anymore. Mom told me he hated his first name, Adolph.

"I hated it because it was an old man's name," he said. "Now I'm an old man, so it fits!"

The remainder of our visit was spent walking and talking. Dad took us to the park, down to the water and up on Savin Hill. He showed us the bridge he used to sleep under before the local outreach service convinced him to accept their help. He pointed out houses where he used to do yard work to earn extra money, prior to his stroke. Dad also pointed out the exact spots where he'd fallen down when he was drunk, stumbling from the bar back to his room. Dad half-apologized for his drinking and tried to downplay it. But the truth would come out a few sentences later, when he'd point to a fence he told us he'd collided with in a drunken stupor, giving himself a nasty gash on his head. Along the way, he'd stop mid-story to say "hello" or "howdy" to everybody that we passed.

In spite of my father's pronounced tremor, he was otherwise in good physical shape and kept active. I learned that he did Tai Chi exercises and had his own little rituals that he practiced along his daily walk to help him with his balance. I was pleasantly surprised by this and saw it as a positive thing, as I've read that regular exercise possibly helps ward off or delay Alzheimer's.

On the other hand, there were things Dad told me that caused me to worry about him. The biggest issue, as I mentioned earlier, was my father's reluctance to receive medical care. Also, I noticed that he barely picked at his food when we had lunch, saying he wasn't a "big eater." Additionally, he told Pete and I he often went two days at a time without sleeping. (Apparently I inherited insomnia from both my mother *and* father, if this condition can, in fact, be genetic.) Also, Dad was private to a fault. I got the impression that he distrusted almost all people. When we were at the group home where he lives, he was always looking over his shoulder, in particular when he was checking his mailbox and when he unlocked the door to his room. I got the sense that my father might suffer a sort of mild paranoia.

Dad's room, while messy, had enough space and bare essentials for my dad to be comfortable. He had a twin bed, a mini fridge, laundry hamper, clothes and even a TV set with a VCR. He didn't have cable hooked up to the television, but he had a bin full of movies on VHS tapes. Dad made us promise not to tell anyone he had all those movies; he feared that if the other residents knew he had them, they'd get stolen.

Amongst my father's meager possessions, he had some mementos from what I call his "yester-life..." the years before he became homeless. He'd saved all the cards and photos that I'd sent him over the years. He even kept the empty cookie tins from goodies that I'd sent him every Christmas. He also had an acoustic guitar that had belonged to his second wife, Pamela. He couldn't bring himself to talk much about her. Speaking of her death, he only commented: "That was hard." I got the impression that losing Pamela is what put him into the tailspin that led to his homelessness. I hope to find out more about her someday, as she must have been quite a special lady.

I presented my dad with a special gift during our first visit. I had scanned a lot of my baby pictures (many with Dad in them) and childhood photographs onto my computer, and then uploaded them to a website where I was able to make a beautiful, hardcover photo book, with personalized captions. Dad really liked that! He especially loved the one snapshot of me taking my first steps. "I remember that like it was yesterday," he said. In the photo you can see Dad's hands letting go of me, ready to catch me if I fell, as I made my first wobbly steps towards my mother, who was holding the camera.

Oddly, when I showed Dad the final picture in the book, the one of him and Mom on their wedding day, he didn't know who it was.

"Is this your wedding day?" he asked, referring to Pete and me.

"No, that's you and Mom!" I told him.

"Oh!" He looked at it again, uncertainly. "I don't see too good."

As for the deterioration of their marriage, he told me that my mother had a boyfriend that she snuck around with.

"That boyfriend of hers was always around," he claimed.

"Who?" I asked, recalling that Mom had no shortage of boyfriends in the 1970s, after she and Dad split up. I ran some of their names past Dad, but none of them rang a bell. Was my mother really unfaithful to my dad, or was this another figment of his imagination, like him thinking he heard me on the radio?

When my parents decided to part ways, Mom was the one to break the news to me. I have no memory of this, but my dad says he'll never forget it. Apparently I, being all of two-and-a-half years old, confronted my father in anger: "Mommy says we have to leave because you were a BAD Daddy!" and kicked him in the shin!

Dad didn't go back out west, where his family was, because "I knew I'd never see you again," he told me. Even though he'd moved to Boston, he consciously chose to remain on the east coast so that he'd still be close to me.

I asked my father if there was anything he needed. He complained he was too hot in the shirt that he was wearing and would like something with short sleeves. Pete and I made a dash for the nearest clothing store and purchased a light-weight, button-up polo shirt. He was so grateful, he changed right into it then and there!

It was the least I could do for him.

Chapter 11

Our Second Boston Trip

Our second trip to Boston took place about ten months later. It coincided with the weekend of our sixth anniversary. This time around, Pete and I knew the city a lot better. We took the Red Line from our hotel to Dad's neighborhood. When we arrived, Dad greeted us, once again wearing a long-sleeved dress shirt and a necktie that had seen better days.

"I had to get spiffied up," he explained.

Alzheimer's had not robbed my father of his sense of humor. He was quick with one-liners and zingers as we caught up on things. When we were walking past the grocery store where he told us he does his food shopping, I asked him: "Is there anything you need while we're here?"

"A Cadillac!" he quipped.

He asked me how I was doing.

"Good," I said. "The job's going great, and just life in general."

"Oh, so you're in the service now?"

"No..."

"I thought you said you were a 'General.'"

(Rim shot!)

As we walked to a nearby park, Dad grabbed hold of my hand. I flashed back to being four years old again. Daddy and I were walking up Pacific Street in Mattituck, on our way downtown to look at toys. I was struck with sadness at how much time had gone by.

Pete, Dad and I strolled to a little park. Walking right ahead of us was a mother and her toddler, a little Chinese girl. Dad pointed her out.

"She reminds me so much of you when you were that age," he said.

At first I didn't catch what he meant, given the difference in ethnicity. But I observed her jet black hair and her little pink dress and I understood. I wondered how many other times over the years, he'd seen similar little girls and thought of me. I watched the child playing on the slide and asked Dad if he remembered taking me to the little playground by the bay in Mattituck. He struggled to think, and finally answered "yeah," but I'm not sure if he was telling the truth.

Catching sight of some chickadees (or sparrows; I can't tell the difference), my father said:

"My mother always used to say 'don't you ever hurt the *pajaritos* (little birds), Junior. All they want to do is sing you a song.'"

He told Pete and I a story about how he'd aimed at such a bird with a sling shot when he was about thirteen, never thinking he'd actually hit it. His aim was right on target. The poor bird fell right over, dead.

"I felt about *this* big," he said, holding his fingers an inch apart.

He went on to tell us how he'd been a real sharp shooter with a sling shot when he was a kid, and how he'd loved the outdoors. Except for the scorpions.

"One time I picked up a gunny sack off the ground and there was a whole nest of them crawling around," he said.

I was very interested to hear all this, because my father had never talked to me about his childhood before.

We talked about Mom some more.

"She was a good lady," he said, his bitterness over "that boyfriend of hers" long gone. "Everything was fine up until her folks got involved."

"Well, Grandpa hated everybody, not just you," I tried to reassure him.

Dad related: "The first time I met him, he told me: 'I don't like freeloaders in my house.' I said: 'what are you talking about? I have a job!'"

So typical of my grandfather.

Oddly enough, Dad did not remember the fact that my mother had remarried.

"This is the first I've heard of it!" he exclaimed, sounding almost angry.

"I thought that's why you left!" I retorted, baffled.

"No," he denied.

I'm sticking to my guns on this one. Dad *had* to have known Mom remarried. He knew she had a new last name, Olmsted, I'm sure of it. Plus, those were years when he didn't have to pay her child support. But I wasn't going to argue with him.

The next day, we picked Dad up to take him out to lunch. He was sitting outside his building, in the little front yard garden with a couple of the other residents. One guy, who Dad introduced to me as Al, was just getting into his car. He called me over to talk to him about my father. Pete kept my Dad distracted in conversation while I listened to what Al had to say. He communicated that my father needed more help than what he was getting at the facility.

"He's... He's *lost,*" Al stated.

"You mean the Alzheimer's?"

"Something like that." But Al sounded doubtful. "I mean, sometimes he's just not *here*. I don't know where he goes. He'll be up and scratching at the TV screen. There's no getting through to him when he's like that. He's just lost. They say they help people here, but they don't really do enough. There's too many residents here and not enough staff. There's a full house now. There's more than they can handle. But your Dad needs more. He's got nothing. I mean *nothing*."

I gave Al my business card and told him to call me with more information, or if anything happened. He said he would.

By the time I returned to Pete and Dad, my father was on guard.

"What was he saying to you?" he demanded.

"Oh, just that you've told him a lot about me and that he also has a daughter that he hasn't seen in a long time. And that he's glad that we came to see you," I replied. Which was all true. I just left out the important stuff.

Dad seemed satisfied by that explanation.

We headed off to our destination, a popular neighborhood restaurant called McKenna's. It was a small place, packed wall-to-wall with customers, so we had a long wait to get a table. When we finally were seated, my father commented to Pete: "You know, I think she's the best-looking woman in this place." I looked around, trying to figure out which waitress he meant. Then I realized he has talking about me! I felt flustered. Neither my grandfather or my stepfather ever told me I was pretty.

Our lunch was well worth the wait. I had a nice, healthy veggie wrap, Pete had a grilled chicken sandwich, and Dad ordered a grilled cheese sandwich with a cup of coffee. Unlike last time we went out to eat, this time my father finished every bite of his meal. Because of his tremor, he had me pour the sugar into his coffee for him. It was such a simple ritual, but it touched something deep inside of me. I wished I could had done this every morning while I was growing up. This could have been a scene from some alternate reality: me and dad sitting at our own kitchen table, in a household that was safe and sound, sharing coffee and pleasant conversation together in a world where divorce... and Alzheimer's... didn't exist.

Even though I had to assist him with his coffee and (lots of) sugar, I thought that his tremor seemed less pronounced than it had been on our last visit. I asked him about this, but Dad said that no, it wasn't any better. He said it was constant. I asked him if medication helped. He said that he'd tried some drug that the doctors prescribed for him. While it relieved his tremor somewhat, the side effects weren't worth it.

"It slows you down. Makes you sleep all the time," he said. Then lowering his voice, he added: "And around here, you can't afford to fall asleep."

I worried about my father's paranoia. It seemed to be getting worse. For instance, in the ten months between our visits, I had to assume that he'd read the letters I sent, because he never answered them. At one time, he had someone else write or type letters to me, but it had been a long while since that happened. I can only guess that whoever was helping him moved away or died, and that he couldn't find another person he deemed trustworthy enough to share his private thoughts with. My father does not have a telephone in his room, so I can't call him directly. It's hard to get a hold of him through his caseworker. Usually I wind up getting Leslie's voice mail, or if I do get Leslie, my Dad has already taken off for wherever it is he goes during the day. This extreme secretiveness is so much a part of my father, but it can be an unwelcome barricade between us.

The more time we spent with Dad that day, the stranger his behavior struck me. He talked about seeing his brother Alex in Boston. "He walked right past me and didn't even say a word to me," he claimed. Then he admitted: "I wouldn't know Alex if I saw him today."

In another unlikely sibling scenario, Dad said that he had heard one of his sisters calling his name from the vacant parking lot next to his apartment house one night. His bedroom window faces the lot.

"She was calling 'Junior! Junior!' because that's what they all call me."

"Which sister?" I asked, feigning belief.

"I don't know," Dad shrugged. "By the time I got to the window, she was gone."

Some his stories sounded like half-truths. For instance, he said he was in the Army, but then talked about how seasick he'd gotten "on the ship to Germany." Given my Dad's age (he was born in 1940), he would have fought in the Vietnamese War, not World War II. I thought maybe he meant that he was part of the U.S. occupation that remained in Germany from the end of WWII until the Berlin Wall was torn down in 1989. However, an online search of military records didn't turn anything up on him at all. Is he reinventing his own history? Confusing himself with his father or his brothers? If I hadn't seen that picture of him in uniform in my Grandma Cordova's living room many years ago, I'd have trouble believing he'd ever even been in the service.

My father said something that caused me to flash back to 1991, when my mother had told my social worker that he'd hit her "for mentioning guns." He claimed that Alex and their father, Adolph, Sr. had been shot. He insinuated it was drug or gang-related. Again… very unlikely to be true.

Other statements he made sounded like harmless fantasies. He pointed out a deli where he claimed to have won $1,000 "seven different times," in the lottery. "But I wound up giving it all back, to buy more tickets," he said.

Other aspects of my father's fantasy world were not so innocuous. Back in his private room, he pointed to some objects that leaned against his bedroom wall.

"Those are my sticks," he said. "Those are for combat. Because you never know who might be knocking at the door."

The "sticks" in question were actually about a half dozen assorted rods. One, Pete recognized as being a bar from a barbell.

Others may have been parts of a fence, or tall garden stakes. I asked my father where he'd gotten these "sticks." He said with a shrug: "I don't know. They just showed up."

I was now concerned that my father, in a drunken stupor or in the throes of a panic attack, might seriously injure someone he saw as an "enemy." What if he thought he was being attacked and speared someone through the neck with one of his makeshift weapons? These were pretty large things for him to have been able to sneak in through the front door and then up the elevator to his bedroom. Apparently, no one kept too close of an eye on the residents, and there wasn't a metal detector at the entrance. I'm sure my dad isn't supposed to have such things in his room. I visited him on a weekend, so I did not get a chance to speak with his caseworker or the house manager about my concerns. Leslie was off, and I didn't see anyone around who appeared to be in charge.

Another thing that worries me is Dad's eyesight. He holds his hand out in front of him when he walks. He says this is because he has double vision and he can't judge how far away things are. His left eye strays way off to the side, probably another repercussion of his stroke. I asked him if glasses would help. He says he had some, but he lost them. I suggested he get one of those chains you wear around your neck that you can hang your eyeglasses on.

"I had one of those. I lost them anyway," Dad said.

Somehow I don't think they're anywhere in his room. I have a feeling he either left them in a bar, or dropped them somewhere along the way back when he was intoxicated.

On a positive note, Dad said that he goes to school in the neighborhood. He just couldn't remember what course he was taking. "Something to do with math," is what he said. Leslie later confirmed that this was true. He goes to school Monday through Friday, and "is quite popular there." I'm glad he does have a social life outside of the bar and the group home.

At the end of our visit, Dad and I exchanged another hug. I told him "I love you." He never says it back to me. It's just his way, I guess.

As I was writing this book, I realized that while I had located him, I am still in the process of "finding my father." He is very much a mystery to me. I tried to think of people who had known my father when he lived on Long Island, hoping they would be able to shed some light on the person that he once was. I thought of Bobby Horton, whose late mother, Mabel, had been good friends with my mom. As I mentioned, she actually dated Dad for a short time after the divorce (even though she was A LOT older than him). It's been quite a few years since Mabel passed away. Coincidentally, I recall that she suffered from either Alzheimer's or dementia in her final years. Before she got ill, I remember her reminiscing to Mom and me years later that he was that he was "crazy as a fox." I hoped that maybe her son Bobby could shed some light on what made her say that. I easily found his phone number on the internet. I was dismayed to learn that Bobby had also passed away, just a couple short weeks before I tried to phone him. If that's not irony, I don't know what is.

The next person I thought of was Dee, who lived next door to my Grandma and Grandpa Newalis since 1970. I'd gone to school with her kids. When Pete and I are on Long Island, we usually pay her a visit. It occurred to me as I was working on this book, that she might very well remember something about my dad. I sent her an email, explaining what I was doing and asked if she had any memories of my dad to contribute. A few weeks later, Dee sent me the following message:

Hi Holly,

Sorry it has taken me so long to answer your email. I have been out of town. Looking forward to seeing you and Pete, whenever you get down here. Delighted you got in touch with your father finally. As far as I can remember he was a very nice, friendly, outgoing person, and loved you to death. Whenever you went on a visit with him on weekends, you came home with tons of presents. I know he was devastated about the breakup with your Mom, and I think your Grandfather had a lot to do with that. Tell him I said "hello", and I am looking forward to seeing you soon.

Love,
Dee

It is hard for me not to be bitter towards my grandfather. Obviously, there was his contribution to the breakup of my parents' marriage. But, there is so much else... I'm not even able to talk about it all. It took me fourteen years after Grandpa's death to visit his grave. I told him I forgave him for the hurtful things he said and did those five years Mom and I lived with him. Perhaps I meant it at the time. However, in the two years since visiting that cemetery, so many more things that had been buried in my subconscious have resurfaced. I am mad at him all over again.

I don't know when, or if, I'll pay Grandpa another visit.

Chapter 12

What Next?

The more I thought about my father after our final visit, the more I suspected that there was something else wrong with him, in addition to Alzheimer's disease. I posted a question on an online message board, describing my father's bizarre behaviors, asking for suggestions as to what might be the underlying cause. I got a variety of answers, ranging from schizophrenia to dementia to "maybe he is seeing ghosts." The reply I honed in on was the following post:

"There may also be a vitamin deficiency which is common in people with Alzheimer's. A thiamine deficiency could cause the delusions. He needs to see a neurologist. In the meantime, tell him to take vitamins."

"When I searched "thiamine deficiency," the symptoms matched up to my Dad's. What's more, I also learned that this condition is often caused by chronic, prolonged alcoholism. The thiamine theory could very well be the answer, I told myself at the time. But what's the solution? How could I ever get my father to agree to see a neurologist? My life seems to be one big irony after another; the latest one being that my father lives a subway ride away from Massachusetts General Hospital, which could offer him much-needed help as an Alzheimer's patient. So many headline-making studies and breakthroughs in Alzheimer's research have come from Massachusetts General! My father's refusal of medical help is akin to a person who is starving to death, walking past the open door of a soup kitchen because he or she is too proud to accept charity. It is both frustrating and heartbreaking for me to watch my father deteriorate needlessly.

Finding My Father

This Father's Day, after my second trip to Boston, I put together a care package to send to Dad, which included socks, a neck-tie, a picture of us together from our most recent visit, some sweets, and two bottles of B-complex vitamins. I wrote a short note to explain this part of the gift:

Dear Dad,

I hope you will take these vitamins every day. They will help you with your memory and forgetfulness. I'd like you to live life to its fullest, with a healthy body and a healthy mind!

Enjoy the other gifts as well. Hope it won't be too long before I see you again!

Happy Fathers Day.

Love Your Daughter,
Holly

I discussed my dilemma with my friend Julie. Julie suffers from Multiple Sclerosis, and has resided at Samaritan Keep Home, a nursing home in Watertown, since she was widowed at the young age of 49. Julie is now in her mid 50s. We became friends through the radio station; she also was a friend of my mother's. Despite her circumstances, Julie doesn't feel a bit sorry for herself. She has a large family that visits her often, and, although she's confined to a wheelchair, she is able to use para-transit services to get out and about the city. I think she leads a fuller social life than most able-bodied people half her age! When I told Julie about finding my father, she was very happy for me. She urged me to make an effort to bring my father here and get him into Samaritan. She said he must have insurance coverage that would pay for it.

If only it were that easy. I can't just uproot my dad from the place where he has lived for the past three decades, where the streets and faces are familiar... especially now, with his reality becoming less clear with each passing day. If he's "lost," (as Al put it) in the neighborhood where he lives, what would it do to him to relocate him to totally unfamiliar surroundings, where he doesn't know a soul, save for me and Pete?

The home where my father lives now is one of thirty-plus similar houses located throughout New England. During our last visit, Pete and I discussed with Dad the possibility of him moving to another of the houses, closer to the New York/Massachusetts border. Dad seemed open to the idea at first, then he went into a spiel about how long it takes to "establish yourself" in a new neighborhood.

"That's what I'm trying to do here," said Dad. "Establish myself."

I was confused as to what he meant by that statement. Dad seems to be a well-known figure in his neighborhood. I asked him how long he has lived in the house where he is now, and he replied: "Thirty years. I was one of the first ones to get in here." I was skeptical that he's actually been there for that long. It was less than thirty years ago that I used to get cards and letters postmarked Brookline, not Dorchester. I contacted the organization and asked when that particular house had started operating. They replied:

Hi Holly:

The House was first established in 1996 by a group associated with St. William's Parish in Dorchester. Our organization took over operations in 2008, welcoming its tenants into our family of 550 permanent housing units.

Finding My Father

Just as I thought. Maybe Dad meant that he was in one of their other homes first, and they later relocated him. Then again, I have come to realize that time passes differently in my father's mind than it does by the rest of the world's calendar.

If Dad did agree to move to northern New York, I'm not sure where the right place for him would be. Unfortunately, Pete and I aren't able to care for him in our home, nor do we have the means to hire a caretaker. I'm not sure a nursing home would be the right answer. He is very independent, and although he can't see well or drive any longer, he is strong, and in good physical shape and enjoys walking all around his neighborhood. There is a long waiting list to get into Samaritan, people who can probably benefit from the facility's services more than my father could. In warm weather months, I often see residents of the nursing home off hospital grounds, motoring their wheelchairs or electric scooters through the farmer's market or at the mall. This is a good thing, for folks like Julie, who don't necessarily belong in a nursing home, but are "stuck" there because their families couldn't take care of them. But in my father's case, it would more likely hurt rather than help him. I cringe, imagining Dad, in unfamiliar surroundings in stumbling out of the tavern on Public Square in Watertown, thinking he was still in Massachusetts, wandering into traffic. Or getting robbed of the few dollars he might have in his wallet by unsavory characters who might pick him out as an easy victim … Somehow or other, I am afraid my father would wind up getting lost or hurt if he moved up here and was allowed the same freedoms that he has at his current residence in Boston.

If my father was somehow able to get a room in the nursing home, would the staff tolerate his drinking binges? I fear that with my father's paranoia and the manic episodes that Al described, they might try to commit him to the psychiatric ward. I don't want to make my father a prisoner. I believe that Dad's most treasured possessions are his freedom and his pride.

My father-in-law, like my husband, is a musician. His band often entertains at Sam Keep and other area nursing homes. I would love for my two dads to meet one day. Both of them are so funny in their own, unique way. I can only imagine how colorful a conversation between these two men might be! Unfortunately, that might never happen, as Pete and I recently learned that my father-in-law has inoperable gastric cancer. We have no idea what tomorrow will bring; different doctors have stated varying opinions on his prognosis. The general consensus, though, is that Old Pete's time with us is sadly limited.

There is also the issue of my father's privacy to consider. I've never met anyone so private and secretive as my dad. He won't even let anyone, other than Pete and me, into his room. (God knows he should at least allow a cleaning lady in there!) If he were to move into Sam Keep, he'd almost definitely have a roommate. Private rooms are for patients with deep pockets, and there is a years-long waiting list, as my friend Julie will attest to. Would my father be willing to share his space with a stranger? Doubtful. Then again, maybe he would be more trusting in a relatively safe place like Samaritan. Not that the group home where he is now isn't safe, but a lot of its residents have battled drug and alcohol addiction and/ or mental health issues. Others may have a criminal history, but are seeking to turn over a new leaf and start a new life with a clean slate. Still, my father might view these men as "dangerous." I believe that most of my father's fears are exaggerated, and some of them not based in reality.

I discussed Julie's idea to try to relocate my father to northern New York with my husband. Pete agreed that Samaritan wouldn't be the best place for him. We looked into other facilities in our area, but the same issues arose: the waiting list, cost and the question of whether or not my father can emotionally handle moving to a new area where he doesn't know anyone. Everything

I've read about Alzheimer's stresses that familiarity and a set routine is what's best for them.

And then there is his drinking. A nursing home staff would not want him going out to bars. Dad's been a heavy drinker since before I was born. I can't see him ever stopping.
Some of you reading this might think that it would be in my father's best interest to get him into an alcohol rehab program. First of all, his alcohol use may have already done whatever damage it's going to do, be it to his liver or his brain. He doesn't drive any longer, so he's not a danger to others. In spite of his health issues (the tremor and his bad eye), my dad is a positive and happy person. Now that he's in his 70s, why should I take away one of the few pleasures he has in life? His years left on this planet are quickly running out, and I want him to enjoy life while he's here. Anyway, it's not like he hasn't had the opportunity before to "get clean." He chose to let alcohol rob him of his marriage, his home and who knows how many jobs. He knows better. When I visit him, he never drinks in my presence and actually makes a point of pointing this out to me. I doubt that if I saw him every day, that he would be on his best behavior. Sooner or later, I'd see what Mom saw.

Another option I had was to go against Dad's wishes and contact his family out west. The most obvious drawback with this, was that my father would be probably be angry with me if I went ahead and did what he asked me *not* to do. Secondly, the family might whisk him out to Utah or Wyoming or Colorado, and I might never see him again. As much as I felt sorry for the Cordovas and the despair that they must have felt over their missing brother/ uncle/ son for so many years, I felt a sense of loyalty and obligation to my dad. I decided that I would abide by his wishes, although I didn't agree with his decisions. There is no reason for him to have to live the way he does, barely scraping by from paycheck to paycheck. A better life for him could be just one long-distance phone call away.

Chapter 13

An Unexpected Twist

After I completed writing *Finding My Father,* and had it published as an ebook, my husband confessed to me that he'd taken it upon himself to contact one of my aunts, Virginia, in Salt Lake City. My first reaction was one of anger. I was upset with Pete for doing this behind my back. This emotion was soon replaced by, for lack of a better word, fear.

It sounds odd feel that way about my own family. They never did anything to hurt me. They in no way ever tried to intimidate me into giving up information on my dad, nor did they try to turn me against my mother. They were welcoming and hospitable the one time I visited them. I'd been so excited to find that there were other musicians in my family (not that I am a musician, but I have written hundreds of songs with just lyrics and melody). I had grown up with relatives who were mostly quiet and reserved, who kept their emotions and opinions to themselves. Grandpa Newalis was the other extreme, spouting hurtful words and never seeing anything any way but his way. Hugs and "I love yous" were rare. While my mother bought me whatever I wanted and told me she was proud of me, she wasn't a communicator like me. There were no heart-to-heart talks or deep, meaningful conversations about life, God or world affairs. Family reunions and big get-togethers were non-existent. Relatives fell out of touch and remained distant.

When I was eight or nine, my mother took me to a doctor's appointment, and the nurse who checked us in looked back and forth from me to my mom and brazenly asked: "Is she adopted?" We looked nothing alike, she being of fair skin with hazel eyes and baby-fine hair, and me having olive skin, brown eyes and thick, jet-black hair. The nurse's rude question started a fantasy in my head that continued for several years. I wished that I really was adopted. I used to fantasize that my real mother was a famous singer, like Deborah Harry from the group Blondie, and that one day she'd decide to take me back. I also wanted to be an orphan. I must have watched the movie "Annie" nine or ten times when it was in theaters in the early 1980s, and read the book over and over. I wanted so badly to be "rescued" from the family I felt didn't love me, and whisked out of the lonely world where I just didn't fit in.

Yet, when the Cordovas opened their arms and their hearts to me so many years later, I turned my back on them. My reasons for doing so are complicated. But none of them are good enough. I had a lot of crap to deal with when I got back from my one and only visit out west back in 1992, with my grandfather, my depression, money problems and troubled relationships. A lot of my grandfather's prejudices were probably instilled in my subconscious as well. I was ashamed of who I was. I also felt I didn't deserve all the love and adoration that was showered upon me by my newfound family. Throughout my life, sometimes to this very day, I've often felt like a "phony," like the nice, happy act I put on for the world is a façade that hides a worthless person inside. It's this attitude that has caused me to pull away from people, keep them at a distance and sometimes push them away from me. I now regret the years I let go by without the Cordovas being there for me and vice versa.

Anyway, getting back to the present; Pete knew I'd been looking up some of my cousins and other members of the Cordova clan on Facebook. I'd shown him their pictures and pointed out the family resemblance. He asked me several times if I wanted to get back in touch with them. I went from saying "no" to "I don't think so" to "I don't know." I guess he got tired of my indecision and waffling. Additionally, he keeps reminding me that we are going to need help with my dad sooner or later. He feels it is too much for us to handle by ourselves.

When he first told me that he'd sent an email message to my Aunt Virginia and had gotten one in return, I told him: "You've opened a Pandora's box."

As usual, I was over-reacting. Since then, I have been very slowly rebuilding my relationship with the Cordovas. At first, Pete did all the communicating for me. Virginia was happy to hear that I was well. She cried when she learned that my mother had died. And naturally, she was overjoyed to learn that "Junior" was alive! My aunt did her best to understand my fears about reconnecting with the family. She certainly understood my worries that I might damage the fragile relationship between me and Dad by revealing his whereabouts and giving up his secrets.

"Holly is our main concern," she told Pete in an email. *When she is ready to deal with all the family, she can be the one to make the final decision on when."*

Cautiously, in small increments, I began to befriend the family... via Facebook, what else? I haven't actually talked on the phone to any of them yet. I have always felt safer keeping a distance from people. I let very few of them into my heart; I've been hurt too many times in my life. The first Cordova relative I started communicating with was a cousin I didn't even know I had, Eleanor. She is the daughter of my father's eldest brother, Henry. I'd met her sisters, my cousins Elaine and Valerie, on that long-ago trip. Other members of the family began friending me as well, including some of my second cousins, who ranged in age from three to eight years old when I met them in 1991... Cierra, Reyna, Andrea, Brittney and Breanna. It was jarring to me to see them now, all grown up and married, some with children of their own. It wasn't until then that I realized how much time had gone by. I wish I had gotten to see them grow up. That's probably my biggest regret about not keeping in touch with the family.

Of course, Virginia and Ernie wanted to be reunited with "Junior." They informed us that many times over the years, they had come close to tracking my dad down, only to have him pack his bags and disappear when he found out they were closing in on him. I can't imagine what he was thinking! In the condition he is in now, it's somewhere between "highly unlikely" and "nearly impossible" for him to pull off another such escape.

Pete put my aunt and uncle in touch with Dad's case manager in Boston. Leslie cautiously bridged the topic with my dad, letting him know that his brother and sister-in-law knew where he was and that they wanted to see him. I don't know how much convincing and cajoling it took, but the end result was a success… Dad FINALLY agreed to talk with them on the phone! Virginia reported back to me that that first, ice-breaker conversation went even better than expected, and that "I love yous" were exchanged.

Even more miraculous, my father agreed to a visit from Ernie and Virginia! (My Uncle Alex, who long ago financed my trip out west, wanted to go as well, but he was too ill.) Virginia invited me to come along as well, but I declined, This was *their* time.

Upon returning from their short jaunt to Boston, Virginia excitedly related the highlights of their trip to me; visiting Boston Commons, taking a bus tour of the city, dining at the famous Legal Seafood restaurant and catching up on thirty-two years of old times with Dad. "He was like a delighted child," she said of my father.

He did not remember my having told him that his parents had died. My aunt tried to attribute this, as well as Dad's short term memory problems, to "just old age." Unfortunately, I believe that is wishful thinking on her part.

As for why he spent so many years running from his family, my father restated his explanation was that he wanted to stay on the east coast in order to be close to me. That's more than a bit baffling, considering he and I never saw each other in all those years that he was living in the area. If I had not tracked him down, we never would have seen each other again, so it wouldn't have mattered whether my dad was in New York, Massachusetts, Wyoming or Utah. It just doesn't make sense. It doesn't explain why he cut his family off. I guess my father has been living in his own version of reality for a long time; the Alzheimer's just makes it that much more confusing for everyone involved.

The happy report of my father's reunion with Ernie and Virginia was soon followed by heartbreaking news; Uncle Alex passed away. A Vietnam veteran, he had been suffering from complications from Agent Orange exposure. He was only 64. I can speak on behalf of the whole family in saying that we're all very sad that he and my father didn't get to see each other again one last time.

My uncle's death has caused other family members to come forward, wanting to visit my dad "before it's too late." At first, there was talk of flying my father out to Utah, which, astonishingly, he agreed to, as long as it was "only for a visit." This would be a challenge, as somebody (probably Pete and I) would first have to fly to Boston to get Dad to the airport safely. We found out from my aunt that Dad has a steel plate in his head from a car accident, so getting him through security could take a long time, as he'd probably set off all the metal detectors! I'm not sure if my father has ever flown. That might be quite the adventure! Pete was worried that the onslaught of relatives might be overwhelming for my dad, but Leslie tells us that since the Cordovas have come back into his life, my father's demeanor has improved immensely. As of this writing, two of Dad's sisters are planning to fly out to see him in Boston soon. This arrangement, reuniting with a couple relatives at a time on his "home turf," makes a lot more sense than trying to fly him out west. However, the clan is planning a family reunion in July, so they might still try to get him out there.

As much as I'd like to attend the family reunion, July is the worst possible month for Pete and I to get away. I already have book signings and another trip booked for that period of time. We can't afford a trip out west just now. Besides, I don't think I can handle meeting all of the relatives at once. I like new things in small doses. I very much want to make a trip to Utah and/ or Wyoming in the near future; I just don't know how or when we're going to make it fit.

In the meantime, I've got to work on my nervousness about meeting everyone again. I look at their pictures and read their Facebook posts and wonder how I'll ever fit in. My myriad health issues make me feel somewhat defective. Namely, the *Neurofibromatosis, which has caused hundreds of tumors to grow all over my body (although the majority of them are on my back and torso, where they can be hidden by clothing). Because of the NF, I decided not to have children, which makes me feel like even *more* of a freak of nature. I might as well be missing a nose or a limb. I especially feel bad about this when I see what beautiful babies my lovely second cousins have. I believe that society looks down on women who choose not to have children, like we must be somehow defective. I have trouble bonding with other women because I feel like we have nothing in common. It seems all they ever talk about is their kids. Most of the time I don't regret staring 40 in the face and being childless, but other times I'm really sad about it, and I wonder "what if...?" Should a cure for NF be found tomorrow, I'd probably still choose to remain a non-mom, but again, this sets me apart from the rest of the Cordovas. I'm barely part of this family, and already I feel like the proverbial "black sheep!"

(*Even though I have a "mild" case of Neurofibromatosis, pregnancy can worsen symptoms, causing my tumors to grow larger and more numerous. Any child I have would have a fifty percent chance of inheriting NF. Common problems from this genetic disorder include bone deformities, facial deformities, hearing and vision loss, learning disabilities, and sometimes cancer. I couldn't live with the guilt of knowingly bringing a severely handicapped child into this world and subjecting it to a life of suffering.)

Then there is the reality of my lifelong depression. It started around fifth grade, when I had the difficulties with my stepfather. Things got worse when we moved in with her parents and I had to endure my grandfather's mistreatment. These were critical years; I was ages eleven through sixteen when we lived there. I was going through puberty. My body was changing. This is a confusing enough time for a young girl. Throw in the fact that my grandfather had no respect for my privacy, and that there were no locks on the doors, and well... you can imagine. I have spent most of my life in therapy and on every antidepressant known to mankind. I know that mental illness is more accepted now than it was ten or fifteen years ago, but there is still a stigma in some cultures. How do the Cordovas view such things? Would they see it as a sign of weakness? An embarrassment? Something to be ashamed of?

Shortly after making contact with my relatives, Pete directed Aunt Virginia to the radio station website so she could see recent pictures of me.

"She's definitely a Cordova!" she told him. "She looks like so many of us!"

Maybe. But you can't judge a book by its cover. I may have similar features, but inside, I'm nothing like they expect. I'm not the 19-year-old kid they met almost twenty years ago. I'm not sure who I am, or what I want.

All I know is I want what's best for my Dad. I hope that whatever decision I make, it's the right one.

Chapter 14

Future Unknown

In the midst of all this change, we are also dealing with the cold reality that Pete's father has inoperable cancer. We learned of this in the latter part of 2010. It's a rare type of gastric cancer. The tumor is in a spot where the doctors can't get at it to cut it out, and so far, attempts to shrink it with chemotherapy have been unsuccessful. He is undergoing chemo and radiation, but one of his physicians have been pretty upfront with the fact that this treatment will simply prolong his life, but the cancer will eventually kill him. The chemo has made him quite ill, and you have to wonder what's worse: the cancer or the treatment? Regardless, Old Pete is going about life as usual, still playing in his band, working in his wood shop and teaching part-time at the college. He has accepted his fate, almost too readily, telling all his friends and colleagues that he is "terminal." My mother-in-law swings back and forth between denial and devastated panic. For Pete and I, it hasn't really sunk in yet.

Naturally, this development has caused me to think about my own dad more than ever. I would love to be able to make it to Boston more than once a year. Unfortunately, our jobs, the economy, our personal budget and the harsh, unpredictable northeast winters do not allow us to travel whenever we please. I hope that Pete and I can visit him again in spring or summer of 2011. A lot of it depends on Old Pete's health.

As for Dad, he seems to be doing well. I think that letting the Cordova family back into his life is the best thing he could have done for his emotional well-being. Leslie says there's a noticeable change in his demeanor. He is still concerned about Dad's drinking, but the Alzheimer's hasn't gotten any worse.

Since learning of my father's condition, I have been trying to learn as much as I can about Alzheimer's Disease. Unfortunately, most of the news out there isn't very encouraging.

Some facts: Alzheimer's Disease is the most common form of dementia. It slowly as the development of plaques and "nerofibrillary tangles" damage and destroy brain cells. More than 5 million Americans, are afflicted, according to the latest statistics provided by the Alzheimer's Association. A recent poll by the MetLife Foundation revealed that Alzheimer's is the second-most feared disease among Americans, after cancer.

There is no proven way to prevent it. While there are drugs to slow its progression, the inevitable truth is that the person with Alzheimer's grows worse over time, starting with short-term memory loss and ending with the inability to recognize loved ones, carry on a conversation, feed themselves or even remember how to swallow. Risk factors include advanced age, family history, cardiovascular disease and race.

My father's Hispanic heritage puts him at a greater risk for developing Alzheimer's than if he were Caucasian. (African-Americans also have a much higher risk than whites.) It is also believed that those who have suffered a head injury have an increased risk of developing Alzheimer's somewhere down the road. I didn't know for certain that my dad fell into this category until recently, when Virginia told us that Dad had been in a car accident long ago, when he was a cab driver in New York City.

Another thing worth mentioning: Alzheimer's is erroneously believed to be "an old person's disease." It's not! At the kickoff party for last year's Memory Walk (which has since been renamed the Walk to End Alzheimer's), all in attendance were shocked to learn that the youngest Alzheimer's patient in the nursing home was only 39 years old. That's my age! That is scary to think about...Alzheimer's is something that could happen to any of us, at any time.

Every day, I scour the news headlines via the internet, looking for new information that might help my dad. Some of the headlines are encouraging: <u>Healthy Diet Could Reverse Alzheimer's Early Effects</u> (from SifyNews.com), <u>Drug Companies to Share Data to Speed Brain Research</u> (from the Associated Press), <u>Heart Study Data Helps Find New Alzheimer's Genes</u> (from MetroWestDailyNews.com), Storytelling Program Improves Lives of People With Alzheimer's (from RedOrbit.com) and <u>Apple Juice Reduces Mood Swings in Alzheimer's Patients</u> (from TopNews.us).

Other are not so hopeful: <u>A Decade Later, Genetic Map Yields Few New Cures</u> (from the New York Times), <u>Alzheimer's Accidental Death Rates Rising In Area</u> (from the Dayton Daily News), <u>Scientists Fail to Link Alzheimer's to Lifestyle</u> (from TopNews.uk) and <u>Panel Finds No Prevention for Alzheimer's</u> (from the Temple Daily Telegram).

There are those that are intriguing, like this one: <u>Protein Links Alzheimer's, Down Syndrome</u> (also from SifyNews.com). This story focused on new scientific findings which found that a protein known as amyloid-beta forms plaques in the brain in Alzheimer's patients, as well as accumulating in the eyes of people with Down Syndrome. Just because doctors discovered this common thread, doesn't mean that they're any closer to curing either condition.

Other headlines are downright weird, such as the New York Post article that claimed that people with beer guts might have a greater risk of developing Alzheimer's later in life. (I would laugh this one off as nonsense, except that they name their source as the Boston University School of Medicine, the same source that produced the study connecting Alzheimer's and Down Syndrome.)

And then there are the sad stories which usually end in tragedy: Alzheimer's Patient Murdered With Morphine in N.C. Nursing Home (from cbsnews.com) and the more recent story about a 91-year-old WW2 veteran with dementia who shot his caregiver daughter in the stomach. I've also seen dozens of headlines about missing Alzheimer's and Dementia patients who go missing after wandering off. Sometimes they are found alive. Sometimes not.

What lies ahead for my dad is anyone's guess. We can't predict how the Alzheimer's will take its course. One thing that's almost certain, is that Dad's future certainly looks brighter for him now than they did a few years ago, thanks to his reconnecting with his family. Whether he lives another five years or fifteen, I want to make sure that the quality of his life is the best that it can be, and that he receives the care that he needs. Even after my dad is gone someday, I'll continue to champion the cause, as it affects so many millions of lives.... Not only of those afflicted with Alzheimer's, but their families and caretakers as well. I hope and pray that sooner, rather than later, Alzheimer's will not make headlines at all, because it won't exist. As you will learn by reading the expert interviews that comprise the last section of this book, we have a long way to go.

But someday, we'll get there.

Holly Gaskin

Photographs

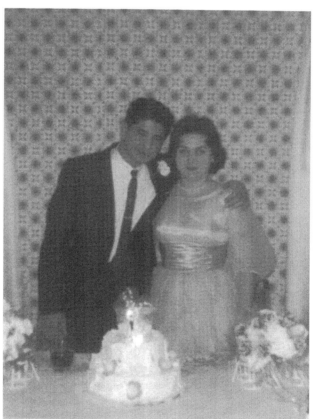

Dad and Mom on their wedding day. I never saw this photo until after Mom's death in 2006. Dad didn't recognize himself when I showed him the picture. He thought it was me and Pete.

Finding My Father

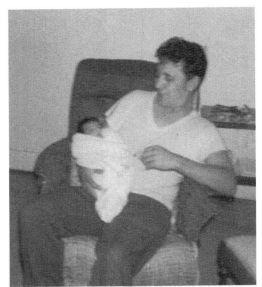

Me and my Dad in 1972. I was two weeks old.

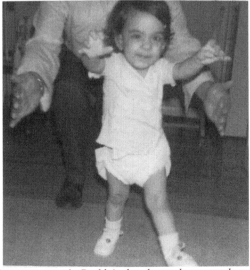

Me taking my first steps, with Daddy's hands ready to catch me if I fell. Even Alzheimer's did not steal this memory from him. "I remember it like it was yesterday," he said of this photo.

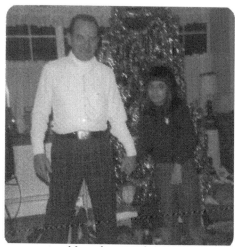

*Me and my stepfather around 1981.
Can you tell I don't even want to be standing near him?*

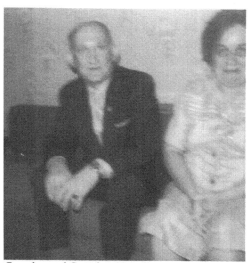

*Grandpa and Grandma Newalis.
My grandfather hated my Dad and wanted me
to have nothing to do with him.*

Finding My Father

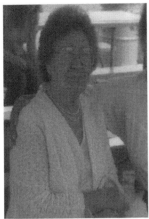 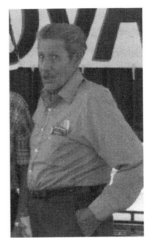

My paternal grandparents, who I met only once. They had been looking for my dad, who they called "Junior," for even longer than I had.

A letter I sent my father in 1997 came back with a glaring "Return to Sender" postmark. I thought he was rejecting me, but he'd simply moved and left no forwarding address.

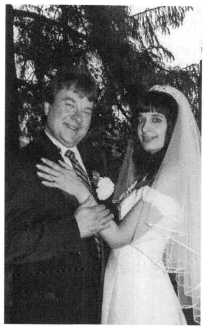

One of the important life events my father missed was my wedding in 2004.

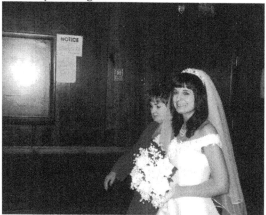

Since my dad couldn't be there to give me away, Mom walked me down the aisle.

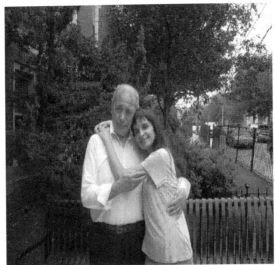
Dad and I in 2009, reunited at last!

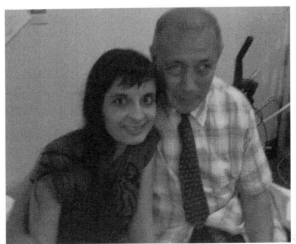
Dad and I in his room. He is wearing the new shirt that I bought him.

Expert Interviews:
Thoughts on Alzheimer's and Elder Care

The following portion of this book consists of interviews that the author conducted with medical and elder care experts via telephone and email over the course of 2010. Information about drugs used in the treatment of Alzheimer's may have changed since then. Many of the statements by the individuals who contributed to this part of the book offered their opinions; none of the following is intended to be taken as scientific fact or medical advice.

INTERVIEW WITH RODNEY RICHMOND, PA

Rodney has been a practicing physician's assistant for more than a decade. He graduated in 2000 from Stonybrook University (Long Island, NY). I interviewed him while he was practicing in Watertown, NY. Currently, he lives and practices in Nashville, TN.

In your practice, do you see patients with Alzheimer's often?
Probably about 1 or 2 a week.

How do you diagnose it?
The only definitive way to diagnose is with a brain biopsy but no-one does that. Mostly, it is a constellation of symptoms that make the diagnosis. Alzheimer's is one (the most common) form of dementia but there are others such as Lewy Body and multi-infarct dementia. Sometimes it is hard to tell the difference. If I am suspicious I look for other causes of memory problems like thyroid disease, infections, inflammatory conditions, strokes and

the like. If these are all ok sometimes I send the patient to the neurologist.

There is a helpful clinical tool called the Folstein Mini Mental Status Exam (MMSE) that I use to help make the diagnosis and follow the progress. This can only be done once in a while or patients will "get good" at answering the questions and confound the test.

Once the diagnosis is made, what are some of the first recommendations you make?

I try to understand the expectations of the patient and family. I try to help them understand what to expect. Many times people feel as if the day the diagnosis is made, life has to change. Usually, that is not the case. When the diagnosis is made, usually a patient has it for a long time. It is important to figure out what is safe and reasonable for him or her and not just assume they have to stop doing certain things. Things like: driving, cooking, traveling, and living alone are examples. I try to look at how they function, what alternatives there are and then try to come up with a long term plan. For example, if the patient still drives, lives alone, handles finances, and functions completely independently, I may recommend a family member just check on these areas to see if there are problems. I will ask the patient how they will know when it is time to give up one or all of these. How will they know? If the patient has some ideas of warning signs, they may help later when these signs appear. Giving up independence is the single hardest part of Alzheimer's on the part of the patient. For the family, one of the greatest challenges is finding time to do all the things the patient can no longer do. I recommend that they all look at the house, apartment, and so on and look for problem areas. Trip hazards like throw rugs and extension cords need to be eliminated. Make sure there is a way for the patient to call for help, probably a cell phone that is with them at all times. If driving is a problem, get rid of the car. Make sure smoke and CO alarms are working.

I ask them to consider alternative living arrangements. If living with a family member is a possible option I try to get everyone thinking about it. If not I try to explain the options such as the difference between nursing home and adult homes.

I also try to help the patient and family prepare for the nearly inevitable conflicts that tend to ensue. Patients usually become very angry and/or frustrated at losing the thing they have relied on all those years, their memory. They often take it out on the people trying to help them overcome this loss. It's very common so I tell both sides, it will probably happen. Help them plan for it.

I advise the family to plan to have backup, time off and such. It is not uncommon for the caregiver to die first, perhaps because they neglected their own health, needs, and so on.

What are the FDA-approved drugs used to treat Alzheimer's?

Aricept, Namenda, Cognex, Exelon and Razadyne. Some companies have studies that show improvement in function through studies like the MMSE but generally these meds just slow the progression of the disease. Many have side effects. it is important for patients and families to have appropriate expectations here as well. If a patient starts a medicine, gets an upset stomach and doesn't see any improvement they may be more likely to stop.

If you were sure an elderly patient had Alzheimer's, but they were in denial and refused treatment, and you thought they might be a danger to themselves... what would you do?
I negotiate as much as I can. Usually I can find some middle ground. If it really comes down to a patient who is at real risk for self harm I can call Adult Protective Services. Interestingly, a patient who has capacity to understand the implications of their decisions, can continue to make their own decisions. It can

become very complicated when a patient who has capacity makes decisions that I don't agree with.

I understand that there is a connection Parkinson's Disease and Alzheimer's Disease.
Parkinson's causes a dementia of its own. It can be hard to tell one form of dementia from another, but the dementia that can be related to Parkinson's resembles Alzheimer's and may respond to medications similarly. Parkinson's disease is "caused" by a loss of the *substantia nigra* in the brain, an area which produces a chemical called dopamine. The loss of dopamine causes the rigidity and tremor associated with Parkinson's. In the case of Alzheimer's a biopsy would show "neurofibrillary tangles" in certain areas of the brain.

I read that Blacks and Hispanics have a higher incidence of Alzheimer's. Does anyone know why?
It is true. Nobody knows why.

If I have a parent with Alzheimer's, how much does that increase my risk of developing it later in life?
Yes, there is an increased risk.

That's all for now... I truly appreciate your input!
Hope this helps.

Holly Gaskin

INTERVIEW WITH PATRICIA WILKINSON

Pat Wilkinson is a retired Registered Nurse. She worked in the Public Health System for twenty years, in Fort Lauderdale, Florida and in Rochester, Syracuse and Watertown, New York.

How did you come to specialize in Alzheimer's?

I didn't really specialize in Alzheimer's. I worked in a nursing home in Rochester for two or three years before I came up here (Watertown), and I worked at the hospital here at Samaritan Medical Center. I worked on a medical-surgical floor, and there were always patients on that floor waiting to transfer over to the nursing home when there was a bed available. A number of them had Alzheimer's Disease, but they also had other medical problems that put them in the hospital. When I left the hospital and went into public health, they had just started a long-term home health care program, which, in New York State, is an alternative to nursing homes. You have to qualify for a nursing home to get on the program. It provides both nursing and social services under Medicaid. We would admit patients who had family at home, but whose family needed respite. We had a contract with Mercy Hospital for their Alzheimer's day care, and Medicaid would pay for it.

You've mentioned that the word "senile" is being phased out in the medical world.

Well, they used to say "senile dementia," which meant the person is old and that they have a dementia. It kind of went along with the thought that it's something that happened to you when you get old, which is not true. It is a disease. It is debilitating. Not everyone gets it when they get old. I've seen some patients in the last six months, like one lady that was 102 years old, and she was sharp as a tack. Every once in awhile we see pre-senile dementia or senile dementia as a diagnosis, but rarely.

What are some tips and tricks people can use to keep their mind sharp as they age?

One of the big things is diet. The same kind of diet you'd eat to prevent heart disease, to keep your heart as healthy as possible, is also gonna help your brain. Lowfat, low cholesterol, lots of fruits and vegetables, easy on the sweets and carbohydrates.

I've heard different opinions from others that I've interviewed about this next question: After diagnosis, what is the average length of time until the disease ultimately claims their life? Or, is there not there an average?

It varies from person to person. Folks can live up to twenty years with dementia. Some of the older folks—which generally happens with any kind of disease—is the older you get, your system kinda slows down and it doesn't progress as fast. So, for folks who get diabetes when they're older, it's not as severe as if you get it when you're young. I think it's the same with things like cancer. You might have a tumor, but it grows slower if you're older.

There are more and more cases of "early onset" Alzheimer's lately. What is considered early, and why do you think this is happening?

As far as I know, there are some people who develop it in their 40s and 50s that we see. That's early onset. I don't know why, other than we're able to get it diagnosed easier and sooner. Years ago, folks with mental illness went to a mental institution, including those with Alzheimer's. Probably about twenty years ago, they stopped taking those with Alzheimer's into mental institutions because the treatments and therapies used for mental illness didn't work on these folks. And they discovered that this wasn't a mental illness, it was a degenerative disease.

The first time I saw you give a presentation, another woman in attendance told a poignant story. She'd witnessed an elderly man in a drug store who was buying a Mothers Day card. Obviously, his mother must have been long since deceased, and the card should have been for his wife. A younger man, presumably his son, was with him, and could not get him to comprehend the situation. You said that it's very important not to get angry or even try to reason with an Alzheimer's victim in this type of scenario. How should it be handled?

There's no sense in arguing with these folks, because it's not that they won't do it or don't want to do it. It's that they can't do it. They can't understand. They, like this man, lost that ability to realize that his mother is gone and it's a card for his wife. So, there's no use in arguing with them. You need to drop it. You need to distract them in some way. Give them something else to do. Suggest they go look at something else if they're in the store. If you're home, and you want them to do something like take a bath and they won't, say "let's go have a cup of tea now." Let things kind of settle down and then work your way back into whatever it is you want them to do. You're not gonna convince them, if they've lost their recent memory, that this is what's what. They don't remember.

You mentioned a phenomenon called "Sundown Syndrome," that their confusion can get worse at night. Can you elaborate?

The symptoms seem to get worse at night, just when the sun goes down. You can start putting on lights in the house, but it's still kind of like, I want to say a "twilight zone." There's that twilight time, where they can't see as well. They see shadows. Of course, we all see the same thing, but in their mind, everything gets more confused in the evening. Keeping the lights turned on seems to help some people. Other people, they're just up all night, and they're calling their family and saying "help," or they're calling the police. They see something that isn't really going on.

What are the final stages of the disease?

In the final stages, they really have no recognition for anybody. They're usually incontinent. That's one of the things that gets them into the nursing home. They can't toilet themselves or feed themselves.

And you mentioned that they forget to swallow?

The swallowing reflex will cease right at the end. It's probably because the area of the brain is affected that controls your swallowing. So they can't communicate, they're bedridden, they're dependent on someone for everything. For bathing, dressing, feeding... all activities of daily living. They can't perform any of them.

Are there any words of hope or encouragement that you can offer?

We need to certainly care for these folks and remember that they are our family members and they are human beings and give them the respect that they need. Try to keep things calm. Try to find a sense of humor in things. If you look, there's a usually a sense of humor, something funny going on here and there. Just take care of them as best you can, and deal with it as best you can without getting upset and frustrated with them, because they're already upset.

And treasure them while they're here.

Yes.

Holly Gaskin

INTERVIEW WITH CHERYL CHOW

Cheryl Chow is a brain fitness and brain-enhancement expert. She is an author writes mostly about medical and health issues. Her mission is to teach her readers how to improve brain health and mental alacrity for better health and happiness. Cheryl's website is www.brainvigorate.com.

What's the definition of "brain fitness"?

I'm not sure there's a definition that everyone agrees on. I think of it very much like physical fitness, only it's for the brain. It's a state of health and well-being.

Now, of course, the brain isn't a muscle, but you can think of it like a muscle. It responds to it like a muscle. "Use it or lose it" applies to the brain as well. So, brain fitness means that one's brain is healthy, and is able to perform its various tasks and functions in an effective manner, allowing one to live a fruitful and productive life.

Brain fitness means not suffering from various illnesses, such as Alzheimer's or mood disorders. Analogous to physical fitness, to attain and maintain brain fitness requires vigilance and adherence to a healthy lifestyle. That means a healthy diet (what's good for the body is good for the brain; and some foods, such as blueberries, seem to enhance cognitive function), regular physical exercise as well as mental exercise, and some type of social support system.

It's been debated whether or not exercise and a healthy diet can help prevent Alzheimer's. So, you are a firm believer in this?

Yes, exercise is a huge component in prevention! Aerobic exercise can cut the risk by 60%. Diet is important, too. Ditto for remaining socially engaged. All these things can make quite a bit of difference -- and they're lifestyle changes that everyone can make.

INTERVIEW WITH DIANE CARBO

Diane Carbo is an Elder Care Expert. She founded the website www.aginghomehealthcare.com.

You say you were motivated to get into the field of elder care because of your grandmother. Did she have Alzheimer's?

My grandmother was given the diagnosis of senile dementia. Looking back, at what I know now, I am sure it was Alzheimer's.

Tell me about the kind of person she was, before and after her mental decline.

My grandmother was a very active individual. She exercised everyday, walked everywhere and was conscience about her diet. She read often and was a whiz at math. She started her mental decline in her late 80s. Physically she was in good health, but her mental status started with confusion, then paranoia. She lived into her late 90s.

Your website, www.aginghomehealthcare.com, has tons of information on home health care for the elderly. Is this a good option for someone with Alzheimer's? Or are they better off in a nursing home setting?

The goal of www.aginghomehealthcare.com is to help individuals to remain at home for as long as possible. Home care is an option for some individuals, but not all.

There are many factors to take into consideration when providing care for someone with Alzheimer's to make a promise to keep someone at home. I believe that the care giver and the aging senior should have a conversation when the diagnosis is given to determine expectations and everyone's limitations. Care-giving is a journey that can last for months to as long as many years. Some may live with the diagnosis for 10 years or longer.

The individual providing the care must understand that providing care for another human being can become an all-encompassing job. That is why, I feel it is important to sit and open the lines of communication to learn what the expectations may be and what the limitations and the boundaries of the care giver may be.

Caregivers may feel that can they can handle anything when the time comes. What they do not realize or take into consideration are nights of interrupted sleep, not being able to eat, feeling run down and worn out. Those feelings come much later. Trust me; feelings of chronic stress, guilt, frustration, and even rage are part of feelings that occur when caring for another.

I believe that putting strategies in place, such as exchanging open communication about expectations and limitations is a good start. In order to for a caregiver to know what their limitations may be, I suggest that you review that stages of Alzheimer's and review what may behaviors may occur at each stage. Incontinence, wandering, aggressive or assaultive behaviors are just a few examples of behaviors some caregivers may not be able to deal with at home. When a caregiver and aging senior with dementia begin to have these conversations, both will come to realize that it will take more than one person to provide care.

I also want to emphasize to care givers the importance of taking care of themselves. IT is important when discussing providing care for your spouse or your parent that you make sure that you the care giver will take time daily/ weekly for yourself. I cannot express to the primary caregiver enough that you deserve a life, and there will be life after this care- giving journey. Your outside relationships will need to be nurtured and developed, as well, if you want a life to return to when this is over.

It is a sad statistic, but it has been found that many seniors with Alzheimer's outlive their primary care giver. Do not take my advice lightly. Utilize a team approach to providing care in the home. If that is not possible, then an alternative setting, such as Assisted Living or Nursing Home should be considered.

What are some of the most common frustrations a caregiver faces with an Alzheimer's patient? Specifically, behavioral problems.

There are many different behavioral problems that the caregiver faces with the Alzheimer's patient at home. Many stem for communication problems. It is important that family caregivers learn as much about the stages of Alzheimer's and potential behavior problems that may occur.

The family care giver needs to learn to focus on the remaining strengths their family member has, not the functions that they have lost. A calm positive approach is always important. A family care giver should investigate and try different approaches to find which one best suit their needs for the different levels of Alzheimer's.

Do most caregivers tend to be family members? Are families reluctant to bring in a professional, such as a home health aide?

I am finding that most caregivers are family members and there is a reluctance to bring in outside help such as a home health aide. Many family care givers have a tendency to think that no one will provide care or do things the way they do.

It is the same feeling a young mother has with her child. A family caregiver must realize and accept that in order to maintain their own physical and emotional health, outside help is necessary. It is so important that the care giver learn to educate, teach and advocate for their aging family member with Alzheimer's to other health professionals from the doctors, nurses and home health aides.

A family care giver needs to realize early in their care-giving journey that this journey will require a team of people. A single, solitary care giver cannot provide care that is required without suffering severe physical and emotional consequences.

Do most insurances, including Medicaid, cover home health care?

I would first like to explain the difference between medical home health care and non medical home health care. Many individuals believe that when they need assistance in the home that Medicare will cover those services. That is a big misunderstanding.

Medicare and HMOs will only cover what is medically necessary. The rules for home qualifying for home care are very clear. In order for Medicare to pay for services in the home, the patient must be home bound. Home bound means that a person is not able to leave the house except for the purposes of seeing the doctor or going to church. There must also be a skilled need. That means that an individual must need physical therapy, wound care or other needs that require a nurse to come into the home several times a week for short visits. Medicare will pay for intermittent visits for a short period of time.

Non medical home care addresses the everyday needs of an individual. These services may vary from being a companion, to light housekeeping to bathing, dressing and feeding an individual.

Community resources such as the Area on Aging and Alzheimer's Association will help you become aware of programs in your area that support in home care. There are many Medicaid waiver programs that provide money and care for individuals that qualify for nursing home care but prefer to remain at home.

There are many religious organizations that offer services and you do not need to belong to any denomination. Check your local listings for the information in your area.

Of course, many veterans' and their spouse have home health benefits available to them that are not utilized. The program Aid and Attendance Program is available and is under utilized by veterans' and their spouses. This is a program that can benefit many in an effort to financially support the efforts to keep some one at home as long as possible.

I have introduced you to the two kinds of home care, skilled and custodial care, but there is a third level of home care that should be addressed here as well.

This third level is hospice care, or end of life care. As a nurse, I feel that the health care professionals wait way too long to refer to hospice. There are many reasons for this delay, which I will not address in this chapter today, but I want families to know that they can call a hospice company and ask them to come out and discuss the services they offer.

Hospice is a choice of how to plan for end of life care. Calling a hospice organization before you need the services will give you an opportunity to understand what is available and how to access these services when the time comes. Many times the family simply can make a call to the hospice company and a nurse will come out and do an evaluation.

After an assessment, if it is an appropriate time and the aging senior meets the criteria hospice guidelines, then a call to the doctor will be made and services started.

For family members with loved on at the end stages of Alzheimer's disease having hospice in early is a blessing. Your care giving journey has been a long, lonely one.

You are exhausted from years of providing care, experienced years of chaos, had years of not having anyone to talk to, or be with. Many of the care giver's of Alzheimer's patients have worked so hard to make a better life for someone who is fading from this one, and is not aware of what is happening. For those family care giver's, hospice will offer support, spiritual guidance and a helping hand on the last part of their care giving journey.

I believe that for the family caregiver's of end stage hospice patients, having hospice started early as important for the caregiver as the patient.

So many caregivers' have socially isolated themselves while providing care and find that they have little or no emotional support at a time when they need it the most. Hospice offers that support the family care giver has been lacking for such a long period of time.

Many caregivers have started their grieving process long before the physical death of their loved one. This gives them an opportunity to work through the grieving process, but helping them realize the transition back into a non caregiver role. Hospice actually offers a bereavement benefit where they will follow up with you for 18 months following the death of your loved one, if you feel you need those services.

If you are a family caregiver that is unsure of a person qualifies for hospice, I would encourage you to call and ask the hospice company to send a nurse out for a free evaluation.

Do you think a lot of the elderly population with Alzheimer's/ Dementia aren't getting the care they need because of lack of coverage?

That is a difficult question to answer. Family members try very hard to keep their senior family member at home, trying to avoid institutionalization. Providing care costs money.
The reality is, the care that is needed is considered custodial care and not "skilled" care in any way. Family members learn about "spending down" and the harsh reality of paying for the cost of assisted living or nursing home gives most family members sticker shock.
I find that many family members try to protect what they consider the "family inheritance".

Many family members have neglected to investigate Medicaid asset protection planning. There are laws on the books that individuals can and should take advantage of, but do not. This is a part of estate planning that many miss. Before I go any further, please understand, this is not just for the wealthy. The average middle class person has access to protect their assets so that everything does not have to go to the nursing home. Of course, it does take planning ahead.

What about home safety for the elderly? What sort of accidents might someone with Alzheimer's/ Dementia be prone to?

Falls, fires, driving safety, medication safety and wandering are the top concerns a family member will most likely have to deal with a family member that has the diagnosis of Alzheimer's.

Is there a safety checklist?

I have an extensive home safety checklist on my site- as well as fire safety checklist. I also have a new product that I will be putting on my site for fire prevention. This is an inexpensive item that actually turns the stove off when you walk away and forget you were cooking. It will be a life saver and give many family care givers peace of mind.

Home safety suggestions:

Beside the recommendations made for basic home changes, the aging adult suffering from Alzheimer's does not recognize obvious dangers.

- In the bathroom, install safety locks on cabinets containing medicines, household cleaning agents, razors and other potentially dangerous items. You can also move these items to a padlocked toolbox or elsewhere.
- In the kitchen, put safety locks on drawers or cabinets containing matches, liquor, knives, household cleaning agents, scissors and any other potentially dangerous items.
- Put safety knobs on your stove, or install a timer so the stove can only operate during certain hours.
- Remove locks from bathroom and bedroom doors. A senior with Alzheimer's might lock a door and then not remember how to unlock it.
- Decorate with solid colors whenever possible. Patterns can confuse someone with Alzheimer's.
- Keep the home well-lighted at night. Waking up in total darkness can disorient an Alzheimer's patient.
- Place additional locks on doors a senior might use to leave the house and wander off. Locate the locks high up on the door or somewhere else difficult for the senior to find.
- Consider a GPS system for wandering patients. They keep track of a potential "wanderer" and gives an instant alert if they leave the area.

- Put solid black mats on the floor in front of doors leading outside. These can appear as deep holes to an Alzheimer's patient and may keep them from passing through the door.
- Check outside the house for potentially dangerous items such as saws, lighter fluid, power tools and paint. Put such items in a locked garage or tool shed.

In addition to home adaptations, keep in mind a few other safety considerations when dealing with seniors suffering from Alzheimer's:

- If you have a smoker, remove things such as ash trays, matches anything related to the activity of smoking. There will come a point, when they will not be able to smoke unattended. You may consider a non flammable apron to place over the aging adult when smoking to prevent burns.
- Some Alzheimer's adults put things in their mouths, so remove poisonous plants and any small objects that could cause choking.
- ID bracelets or necklaces containing medical information and a phone number should be worn at all times, if you don't have a GPS system or a medical alert system in place. It is important to be able to identify the aging adult and locate the family should they wander from their home.

Any closing thoughts?

It is important for seniors to stay engaged and involved in activities of interest to them for as long as possible. Because the illness follows a different course in each individual, it is part of the caregiver's responsibility to continually reassess the situation and determine when a senior can no longer safely perform a particular function.

INTERVIEW WITH RICHARD TAYLOR, PH.D

Richard Taylor is a retired teacher and psychologist, who was diagnosed with Alzheimer's in 2002. When the disease made it impossible to continue working, he retired and began traveling the world, as a public speaker, advocating better care for those living with a diagnosis of Alzheimer's and other forms of Dementia. Richard is the author of <u>Alzheimer's From the Inside Out</u>. At the time I spoke with Richard, he had just returned from New Zealand.

Richard, how many speaking engagements do you do per year?

I'm on the road maybe two or three weeks out of the month.

The reason I'm writing my book is because I found my father after 30 years of separation, and he's in the early stages of Alzheimer's. But I think there could be other stuff going on as well. I think he may have some brain damage as a result of decades of alcohol abuse. Some of his symptoms aren't consistent with Alzheimer's, like when he gets paranoid and delusional.

Well, there's the probability of frontal lobe dementia, too.

What's that?

There's about fifty different forms of dementia. Alzheimer's is just one of them. There's really not much you can do for it, one way or the other. If it's alcoholism, stopping drinking certainly will help.

I think it's a bit late for that. Also, we don't live near each other. I'm in upstate New York. He's in Boston,

Massachusetts. He's free to come and go as he pleases, in his group home. Unfortunately, most of the coming and going involves trips to the bar and back.

Now, you mention in your book that when they first made your diagnosis, they did a lot of unpleasant testing. You mentioned a spinal tap and taking lots of blood. Is that normal, when they're just trying to diagnose Alzheimer's?

Not a spinal tap, but they try to rule out all the reversible forms of dementia. To do that, they have to do a lot of different blood tests. They'll probably take a CAT scan or a PET scan, which are non-invasive. Your dad probably needs that, just to see if there is actual physical damage to his brain from his drinking.

Is there an official memory screening test that can pinpoint Alzheimer's?

No. There is no consensus about how you diagnose it.

There are about five different drugs that can help slow the progression of Alzheimer's, is that correct?

Well, there are three of them that are very closely related to each other. They're virtually the same drug. Aricept, Exelon and Reminex. (AUTHOR'S NOTE: I think Richard meant Reminyl; Reminex is a pill that supposedly fights gray hair.) In thirty to sixty percent of the people that take them, it may slow the progression of the disease. But we don't know what the progression of the disease is in any one individual. There's no dramatic changes, usually in people.

Do you take anything?

Yes, I take those, and another one called Namenda. It's a European Parkinsonian drug. But none of them really... I think we'll look back in ten years and say "what a waste of money that was."

In the beginning of your book, you say that your whole ordeal started when your daughter cam home to visit and she took your wife aside and told her, "something's wrong with Dad." What made her say that?

Little changes in my personality, getting lost once with her, not going to the doctor once when I was supposed to, searching for words... She'd never seen me searching for words before.

Your book, <u>Alzheimer's From the Inside Out</u> was published in 2006. How much has changed since then?

It's been very slow. It's mostly an increase in the things I just mentioned. Occasionally, when I'm very tired, I have some aphasia problems. I can't get the words out. I have almost no attention span. I just constantly interrupt myself.

Are there any mental or physical exercises you do to help you?

Physical exercises help everybody. Low blood pressure helps everybody. Just being healthy helps everybody. But there's no evidence to say those brain exercises are generalizable to Alzheimer's. There are some that work for strokes, when they can pinpoint a certain area of the brain, but dementia seems to be a generalized disorder of the whole brain. While it increases people's energy, attention and focus, which is fine, there isn't any evidence to say that there's a physiological change as a result.

You said in your book that you've lost hope in new scientific "breakthroughs" in Alzheimer's research. Do you have any faith in any recent discoveries?

Actually, I've become very angry about the disproportionate way that they spend money on research. They spend almost no money researching how to help people with the psycho-social issues of how to deal with Alzheimer's. They keep crying for more money, faster, to find a cure for it . There's no consensus that there is really a disease called Alzheimer's that's curable.

I suppose it's hard to cure something if you don't know the cause of it to begin with.

Exactly. It is a chronic condition. It's something like arthritis. We have some ideas what causes arthritis, but we don't know how to stop it, and we don't know why some people get it and other people don't. There's some things you can do with the condition to make your life easier. That's what dementia is. It's progressive. So is arthritis. There's lots of chronic conditions that human beings have that we just don't know why we have them, and we don't talk in terms of 'we've got to spend a billion dollars to cure it.' We focus on, how can people have a quality of life when they have it. There's very little on that focus.

Do you advocate the Memory Walk and those type of fundraisers?

No. The local chapters, yes. The local chapters do a yeoman's job of trying to educate people locally. The national chapters spend sixty cents of every dollar on looking for a cure.

Back to your personal life. You mentioned in your book that people kind of talk around you. Like, if you're with your wife, they'll ask her questions about you, that you could answer, like you're not even there. Is that still happening?

It's worse over time.

That must be frustrating.

It is very, very, very. It's even more frustrating now, because sometimes they're right! They never used to be right. But it's still frustrating.

How about depression? Do you suffer from depression?

It comes and goes. I get on antidepression medicine for six months and then I wean myself off of it. Then I get back on it. I don't like messing around with brain chemistry when we don't understand what causes depression.

Do you still feel, as you said in your book, that you're existing in a purgatory?

No. I'm pretty well convinced that I have dementia. What type it is, I have no idea, and I've lost interest in finding out. I know it's not some types, because I've met people with those types. I know it's not vascular dementia. That can be seen in a CAT scan. I know it's not frontal lobe dementia, because I don't exhibit those symptoms. I just see it as some sort of generalized dementia. I don't need a word, because there's no different treatment for whatever word you use or whatever your condition is.

Who is there for you in your daily life, besides your wife? Do you have a caregiver?

Uh-huh. I have an assistant. She stays with me most of the time when my wife is not with me.

You must close your speeches with something positive, or words of hope.

Well, I don't have words of hope. I have words of reality that we need to live in today. We need to use the reservoir of love that we have to make today as rich as possible, and then deal with tomorrow when it comes. I think hope drains people's positiveness. First of all, it says to people, "today is awful, but tomorrow might be better.," when we really don't know what tomorrow is. I've got a higher probability it's not going to be better than yours is, but we both need to live in today. And today is what I have trouble understanding, so I have to even live in today more than you do. You can wander into yesterday and back into today, and into tomorrow, but I get all mixed up.

Some great words. I really appreciate you sharing your insight with me. I can't wait to share it with a lot of people in my ebook. I'm so glad you're a part of it. Thank you for agreeing to this interview.

You're welcome.

INTERVIEW WITH STANTON O. BERG

Stanton O. Berg maintains the website www.JuneBergAlzheimers.com, which he founded in honor of his late wife. I had some questions about his experience losing both his mother and his wife to the disease, and he kindly agreed to answer them. I expected some brief, matter-of-fact answers, not the detailed account of their wonderful love story. I thought about editing it down for brevity's sake, but I decided to leave things pretty much as Stan wrote it. I know you'll be as touched by his and June's story as I was!

Tell me how you and your wife first met.

My father Tom first introduced June to me. I was home on leave for two weeks from the Army during the time of the Korean War. I was serving in the Army Counter Intelligence Corps at the time. Train travel then was the most common and I had gotten home late the night before on the train. It was a two day travel from the Counter Intelligence Corps. Center in Baltimore, MD where I was stationed. So bright and early on Tuesday morning the 22nd of May in 1951, my father Tom took me down to meet this "special lady" that worked at the café where he always had his morning coffee in the little town of Barron, WI. I really was not interested in going to meet some girl because I had my own ideas of girls to connect up with. But I did not want to hurt his feelings so I went along with him. Well, that meeting changed my life forever. I have often wondered if this was a divine appointment.

June and I had coffee that evening to get acquainted. We then made plans for our first real date the following evening (Wednesday the 23rd of May, 1951) at a little restaurant called "The Spot" located on the connecting narrows between two small lakes at nearby Chetek, WI. We had dinner there and walked by the lake afterwards and talked and made plans to see each other every day for the remainder of my leave time. I remember June saying the steak she had that night was her first ever steak.

We were both children of the "Great Depression" and as such had lived a rather frugal life. We were both the poor families in our respective farm areas where we had lived. World War II came along and ended the Great Depression by offering full employment in war industries or in the service. June and I were just starting high school when the war started. When we graduated from high school WWII had just ended. Because the selective service draft was still in operation and I expected to be drafted to provide occupation troops for Germany and Japan, I enlisted in the Army in the spring of 1948. I enlisted for three years in order to be able to pick my branch of service and specialty area. Of course when the Korean War came along on the tails of WWII, Congress was kind enough to extend my enlistment (by a bill in congress) from 3 years to 4 years in order to maintain troop strength. I served my time and was discharged in May of 1952.

June and I were engaged on Tuesday, November 13th, 1951. I had taken a 16 day leave from the Army in November to visit home and see June. I arrived home in Barron (via train) late on Monday evening the 12th. I met with June on Tuesday the next day when I proposed and she accepted. My first ring for June was rather small but she acted like it was really special. I could not afford much from my Army income of $125. a month. I remember buying it on time at a jewelry store in downtown Baltimore. We later called it a starter ring. Several years later we replaced it with a much nicer and larger ring. We replaced it again for our 30th anniversary with a still larger and nicer ring. I now wear June's final ring on a necklace around my neck. I had a large man's diamond ring that I removed from my hand and placed on June's finger at her funeral. That ring remains with June at her final resting place in Lakewood Cemetery in Minneapolis.

Finding My Father

June and I were married on August 16, 1952, in Bloomington, Illinois, where I was finishing up a training school for my new job with State Farm Companies. June came down to meet me on the train in Bloomington, arriving on a Saturday morning. Illinois required blood tests to rule out sexually oriented diseases, plus we needed a license. All city and county offices were closed on a weekend. The kind people in Bloomington opened the county/city office just so they could issue us a license. They also rushed the blood tests through. I had made arrangements with a local minister at a Methodist church to marry us on Saturday afternoon. A little old lady living in a large Victorian house moved out for the week to let us take over her home during that first week of our marriage. Looking back and comparing today's mentality, I can hardly imagine such kindness and compassion by so many for a young couple getting married. We were both age 24 at the time.

How long were you married?

June and I were married for 56 years when Alzheimer's took her away from me on Thursday morning October 23rd, 2008 at 7 AM.

How many children did you raise?

June and I raised four children. We have two boys and two girls. David is the oldest, Daniel is next and then the two girls followed. Our oldest daughter is Susan who now lives in Cary, NC with her son and our grandson Daniel. Our youngest daughter Julie lives in Columbia Heights, MN

We have 10 grandchildren and 7 great grandchildren.

What kind of person was June before the Alzheimer's struck?

June was a very caring and loving person. June was beautiful inside and out. The daughter of one of June's favorite cousins was asked by her mother if she remembered June. Her reply was that June was "the lady with the friendly smile and kind eyes!" June was raised on a small diary farm in rural Dunn County, WI by a loving Christian father and mother. June was a very humble lady who never strayed far from the farm girl I first met in 1951. She was without guile or pretense. When I think back over our many years together I find it hard to recall a single cross word that she had for me. June was totally unselfish and always placed all who were close to her before herself. She lived an exemplary life with a strong faith in God. Through her church, Redeemer Lutheran (member for over 50 years) June performed many services for others. (Girl Scout Leader, Sunday School Teacher, delivered "Meals on Wheels," was a nursing home volunteer, served on her church board etc.) She gave little importance to her own accomplishments. To me June has been a lady for "All Seasons". A very unique, bright and highly principled Christian lady. While June like everyone has likes and dislikes, I have never found her to be uninterested or bored with any thing that life has presented her. June was well traveled. She traveled to Europe eleven times and made at least 100 trips in and around the U.S. in connection with my forensic matters. June was my Administrative Assistant in my forensic consulting business. June would be included in Tom Brokaw's "The Greatest Generation." She truly made my life an adventure. I once wondered if she could really be an angel on earth, but I guess Angels would not come down with Alzheimer's and would not be married to mere mortals.

What were the early signs of Alzheimer's with June that you noticed first? How old was she at the time?

I hardly saw any early symptoms. June was the one that was concerned about her short term memory, in 1997. I really did not notice that much of a change. It was not that obvious to me. I just thought that she was overly concerned about the normal memory problems that everyone experiences from time to time. In December of 1997, when we had our yearly physical examination by a Doctor of Internal Medicine, June brought the matter up. This doctor gave her some simple memory tests and then told her that what she was experiencing was not normal. He then made arrangements to have June tested at the University of Minnesota in their Neuropsychology Laboratory. Their report, dated 1/26/98, stated that June's intellectual and executive abilities were grossly intact as well as her motor abilities but that there was fairly severe recent memory impairment. This pattern of deficits was said to be most consistent with early stage Alzheimer's disease. Their Alzheimer's diagnosis was later confirmed at Mayo Clinic. Short term memory is of course the hallmark first sign or symptom of Alzheimer's.

How did you and she react to her diagnosis?

I can best answer this question by quoting my letter to our (20 June 1998) children advising them of June's Alzheimer's diagnosis. I resorted to sending them a letter because I knew that I could not discuss it rationally with them without breaking down emotionally and being unable to speak.

"Mom was in for examination in connection with her neck arthritis on Thursday the 19th with Dr. Stein. He commented about the results of the University testing in a rather abrupt manner, assuming we already knew the results. Unfortunately we did not. In any event, we were both shocked and dismayed to learn that the evaluation concluded that Mom is in the early stages of Alzheimer's disease and that she has mild symptoms at this time.

Mom initially seemed stunned and momentarily depressed. However, after a short time that same day, she started cracking jokes with a psychical therapist who was fitting Mom with a soft neck collar in regard to her arthritis symptoms. Mom has not discussed the subject since.

In any event, I am taking this means of advising you, because I think that you as the immediate family members and Mom's children should know, and because I am unable to verbally discuss it calmly with you at this time.

I only ask that you be considerate of Mom and patient with her when she seems not able to recall something that you may have recently discussed with her. Her long-term memory however, seems to be good and better than mine. She frequently can recall happenings of many years ago that I need help in refreshing my memory. I would assume that if Mom wants to discuss this matter with you, she will bring up the subject in conversation. Mom does not know that I am bringing this sad news to your attention at this time.

I feel that this information, at least for the time being, should be kept confidential among the immediate family and not be passed on to the grandchildren or other relatives. Lastly, keep in mind that overall, Mom's Alzheimer's is only in initial/early stages and the symptoms are mild. Hopefully it will be years before any real serious symptoms surface."

Later in a letter to relatives and friends in May 2001, I stated: *June does not mention her AD very often. Unfortunately, I cannot look at her without thinking about it. I still have trouble discussing it. She says that she tries to put it out of her mind. She seems to do relatively well at accomplishing this - or so it seems. Of course no one but June would ever know how well she puts it out of her mind. Some time ago, as we were on our way to one of her class reunions in Colfax, we drove through North St. Paul on 694. June commented that her life had really changed. She made reference to how she in the past, would drive to North St. Paul (or anywhere else in the cities) on personal errands that she now does not feel comfortable doing. On another occasion she commented that she supposed that someday she would have to be placed in a nursing home. When we are out with friends and someone mentions AD or jokes about it, I cringe. June acts as if nothing happened and will ask a question or two and go on. I would think that at times it would be terrifying for her to contemplate life's path in the future."*

June knew at a very early date, the blackness and the depth of the distant approaching Alzheimer's storm clouds. June displayed a concern for me. I remember well that Sunday (1999) when June brought home the "Care Notes" pamphlet from our church - "Handling Grief as a Man." June said nothing; she just left it out for me to find and to read. I remember the time that June detected one of my episodes of emotional sadness as I watched her illness progress. June tried to console me by saying "Don't worry, I will be alright Stan!" I am sure at the time, June and I both really knew otherwise.

What type of treatment did she receive, and do you feel it was helpful as far as slowing the progression of the disease and improving her quality of life?

As most authorities would agree there is no effective medical treatment for Alzheimer's. Nothing by way of medicine or drugs slows the progression of Alzheimer's and very little improves the quality of life for a few and not at all for others. In my opinion, the best treatment for the early and middle stages is simply a loving and caring and understanding environment provided by a loving, caring and patient caregiver. Our regular doctor was a doctor of internal medicine and geriatrics. He prescribed the usual standard approved medication which at that time was thought to be Aricept along with vitamin E. This was later approved by Mayo Clinic.

June started taking Aricept in August of 1998. This was just a few months after her diagnosis of early stage Alzheimer's in January. June continued taking this drug up until November 2004 (6+ years). Her dosage was 5 mg's twice a day. I was never able to determine if Aricept was actually helping June either by improving her cognitive symptoms or slowing the progression of the disease. (Based on the large scale UK study of Aricept, it was most likely of no benefit to June.)

I thought June was tolerating the drug well but as I found out later, that assumption was incorrect. I was afraid to take her off of the drug in the event it was helping her. The decision to remove June from Aricept came as a result of a recommendation by a doctor at the University of Minnesota's Orafacial Pain Clinic. Shortly after June started taking Aricept, she developed facial pain along the left side of her nose and on up to her forehead. At times it seemed to center itself over her teeth. The pain seemed to be intermittent and varied in intensity and at times caused June much distress. Because of the symptoms no one associated it with the use of Aricept. June was seen by two different EENT specialists, the Fairview Pain Management Center and finally by the University of Minnesota Orafacial Pain Clinic. The university gradually ruled out all the various possibilities and finally centered on the Aricept. Such pain is not listed anywhere as a side effect to that drug. Immediately after June discontinued the Aricept, the pain went away forever.

June's Experience with Namenda. This drug was approved by the FDA in October 2003 for the treatment of moderate to severe Alzheimer's disease. It was the first such drug approved by the FDA for this level of severity of the disease. (This drug was actually developed 20 years earlier in Germany and was already in common use throughout Europe.)

June was started on the drug on 10 March 2004. She began a dosage of 5 mgs that was increased in 5 mgs increments weekly until the target dosage of 20 mgs was achieved. (10 mgs twice daily) June seemed to tolerate the drug without any apparent side effects. June continued on this drug until it was gradually phased out and discontinued 4/6/2006. (2 plus years.) It was gradually discontinued after June's Alzheimer's had progressed to the late stages of the disease and June was then in Hospice Care. There appeared to be no reason for June to continue with the drug. I was never able to note either temporary cognitive benefits from the use of this drug or any apparent slowing in the progress of the disease. Her progression of the disease actually slowed down more after she was removed from this drug and all such drugs.

There were a few months of overlapping coverage in the usage of both Aricept and Namenda. (March to November 2004.) No apparent benefit could be noted in June's usage of this drug or the combination usage of Namenda and Aricept.

June's Experience with Depakote: This drug was approved by the FDA primarily to treat seizures and convulsive disorders. It was also being studied as a treatment for Alzheimer's. Some initial research indicated that it had value for such treatment.

June had 4 seizures during her journey through Alzheimer's. The first two seizures took place a month apart in mid 2005. 5/2/2005 and 6/2005. The third seizure took place on July 4th 2006. The last seizure described as a mild one took place in mid year 2008.

I requested that June be placed on an anti-convulsive drug immediately after the first seizure. I pointed out that seizures while they were not considered an everyday Alzheimer's symptom they were not uncommon with this disease. (June had been taken to the nearby hospital emergency room to check out possible brain tumors etc.) Based on the opinion of the emergency room doctor, the first seizure was not taken seriously and was thought to be an anomaly not a part of the Alzheimer's disease. I did not agree but having no medical credentials, my opinion was ignored. When a second seizure took place a month later, June was immediately placed on Depakote.

June was started on an initial dosage of 250 mgs of Depakote. In order to reach what was considered to be a "therapeutic level" (50-100 mcg/ml) in the blood stream, June was given gradually increased dosages by increments of 125 mgs until she was receiving 625 mgs per day. This 625 mgs daily dosage was then continued until June passed away on October 23rd, 2008.

This medication appeared to be very effective in preventing seizures. The first seizure following the prescription of Depakote was just over a year later on July 4th 2006. It was my thought that there had been a breakdown on the administration of the medication that caused the July 4th seizure. June due to her advanced Alzheimer's was difficult to feed and administer medications. Not all LPNs assigned with this function were adept to doing so. It was usually mixed with other foods to facilitate the administration. Some of the medication is always lost in this procedure. It is also my thought that this may have been the cause of the mild seizure in 2008. Sometimes there are errors in medication administration. I recall on one occasion when a new duty LPN had administered the morning medication with an improper dosage. I happened to be there at the time, and I suspected that there had been an error. When I questioned the LPN about it, I found she had administered a single pill of 125 mgs instead of 5 - 125 mg pills to give the proper dosage of 625 mgs. If I had not been there to double check, the error would have gone unnoticed

June was also on an anti-depressant (Zoloft) for several months as a supposed cure for sadness and crying. This was done on recommendation of the first Alzheimer's facility that June was in during 2005. It was of no benefit. I learned later that NO drugs are approved by the FDA for use in Alzheimer's or other dementia diseases.

You had the misfortune of losing both your mother and your wife to Alzheimer's, one year apart. Who was stricken first?

June was the first to be stricken. (Diagnosed in January 1998) During the early stages of June's journey through Alzheimer's I had noted that my mother was having difficulty with her check book and her memory.(2002) Her personal cleanliness in her apartment was starting to suffer. My mother lived in a small town in Wisconsin (Barron) approximately 100 miles away from my and June's home. My mother was born in this small town and lived in it for almost 100 years by the time of her death. She had been living independently for several years in a senior housing development. I noted the parallels in some symptoms and suspected that my mother was also in early stages of Alzheimer's. After it became necessary that I take over her finances and because of her advanced age (94-95) and other health concerns, in late 2003 I arranged for my mother to be in the care of a local assisted living home. Following a fall and pelvic fracture my mother was moved to the local nursing home for full time care. I arranged for an evaluation by a Dr. of Psychiatry as I was sure Mother had Alzheimer's. This medical examination confirmed my own diagnosis. She was officially diagnosed as of 22 January 2004. This then qualified her for Medicaid. June at this point was in middle stages of her Alzheimer's. Mother remained at the Barron Nursing home until her death on October 21st 2007. My mother was just less then two months from her 99th birthday when she died. (Most of her brothers and sisters lived to an advanced age.) It had only been a little less than 4 years since her diagnosis. I think that her advanced age contributed to her shorter life span after diagnosis. Also a significant factor was improper medication by the staff of the nursing home. They were using an antipsychotic drug that was not approved by the FDA for use in Alzheimer's or dementia cases and in fact contained a black box label warning. I was able to get an investigation done by the Governor of Wisconsin that resulted in citations against the nursing home but that did not bring back my mother. At the time of her death, my mother appeared to be in much better condition than June and one could have conversations with her and normal communications.

Was it more difficult to deal with your wife's Alzheimer's than your mother's?

I was far more difficult to deal with my wife's Alzheimer's than my mothers. First, of course, is the fact that my wife was the first to come down with this disease and had the disease for almost 11 years. (My mother had it for approx. 4 years.) Also a factor was of course the close daily relationship that existed between my wife and me. The distance away from my mother was a complicating factor. This small town in Wisconsin was the local county seat and did have a number of medical facilities available and in particular had a number of facilities devoted to the aged. June and I would make frequent trips to see my mother. At some of the critical times (while June was in her early stages.) June and I would make 2-3 trips in a weeks time to look after my mother. I had a routine of calling my mother almost daily. Of course as June's Alzheimer's advanced and after June was in a facility it was more difficult for me to make my visits to my mother. I would usually do so on a Saturday, driving down early in the AM and spending the day with her and coming back to my home that evening. On that Saturday our son David would spend time with June and feed her the noon day brunch. I had established a visitation schedule that provided for a family member to be at June's facility every day of the week. I would be there with June most of the time and was spending 32+ hours a week during the last years. Three of the days were normally covered by our two sons (David and Daniel) and our youngest daughter Julie. Our oldest daughter lived in North Carolina so was not a part of the weekly routine.

Were you your wife's sole caregiver or did you have help?

During the first seven plus years I was the sole caregiver, and during that time June remained in our home. During the later part of the 7th year and early into the 8th year, June started having hallucinations and did not recognize me at times. During such times some of our grandchildren (Gretchen and Steven) would stay overnight as a calming influence. I had to have a much delayed complete right hip replacement surgery in the early part of the 8th year. (February 2005) Our daughter Susan came home from North Carolina and stayed during my week of surgery and recovery. My local youngest daughter Julie would also help out as needed. Our two local sons David and Daniel were called on when needed. It reached a critical point in early 2005 and a decision was made to obtain assisted living facilities specializing in Alzheimer's care to provide consistent care. On 16 March 2005 June became a resident in such a facility. (The Wellstead of Rogers.) A year later I became dissatisfied with the Wellstead. June was transferred to a nursing home that specialized in Alzheimer's care. (The Benedictine Health Care Center of Innsbruck.) This facility was located only a mile from my house Once June was in the care of an Alzheimer's facility; the visitation program outlined above was placed into effect. On the 4 days of the week that I scheduled myself to be with June were days that I arrived at the facility at 9:00 AM and did not leave until 5 PM of that day. I would feed June her Noon brunch and her afternoon snack. I would also take her down to the facility Chapel for prayers and quiet times. June was unable to walk during most of 2006 and not at all for the remaining 2 years time of her life. I would move June about in her Geri chair as needed. While June was having her afternoon nap, I would remain on premises, reading and having coffee until time for her to be awakened. I did not leave for the day until I was certain that there were adequate and competent caregivers on the staff to feed June her evening meal. I had standing instructions that if the staff was unable to properly feed June, I was to be called to come over and do so.

In the beginning I was the only one who could always feed June. I had devised my own method, technique and procedure to do so. I actually trained some of the personnel on how to do this. In late stages the victim of Alzheimer's will not always open their mouth to accept food. They require pureed food and frequently may have problems with swallowing. Later some of the personnel developed their own procedures and some became better and more competent than I was. I also had instructions that in case of any problems relating to June I was to be called. On one occasion in early evening, I received a call that June was having long coughing spells. I immediately went to the nursing home and spent the rest of the evening comforting and assisting June until 2 AM when the coughing abated and June was able to sleep. It turned out to be a condition set up when one of June's medications (liquids) was not administered and swallowed properly so as to get into her lungs. It took hours to clear. We then arranged to substitute the liquid for a dry pill in the future and thereby avoided any repeat of this situation.

How did you get through the difficult years of 2007 and 2008?

During these years June rarely ever opened her eyes and was nonresponsive to speech or any communication. These were very sad times. June did not talk, did not smile and would rarely ever look at me or anyone. Of course during this time, June was unable to walk and rarely even moved her arms. It was difficult to get her to open her mouth for feeding her food or drink. June required total care for her survival. I simply kept on doing my normal daily routines – there were no alternatives. I would hold her hand. I would play some of her favorite music. I would take her to the Holy Spirit Chapel. I would quietly talk to her and tell her I loved her and would always love her and take care of her. I did a lot of praying for June, hoping for a miracle but not really expecting one based on the history of this terrible disease. This is the part of the disease that most people are unaware of. Most would tend to think of Alzheimer's only as a memory problem. June's room was decorated with pictures and favorite items from our home. If June should open her eyes or look around, I wanted her to see something that might be comforting. I also had a small cross located directly in line with June's eyes as she lay on the bed. If she were to wake up at night and be afraid, I hoped she would see God's cross and not be frightened. I required that June's head and shoulders were to be elevated so as to minimize any chance of choking should she cough up fluids. I had a small CD player on the night stand by June's bed. I would start it playing some of her favorite music a little before she was to be awakened from her nap. I also arranged to have it played in the evening for her after she had been prepared for the night. I am afraid that I did a lot of crying in those days. Because Christmas was June's favorite holiday (she used to say she wished it came twice a year), we always arranged to have Christmas Eve as a family affair with June at the nursing home. We would use the family room; have food and music with June in the center of activities. We always hoped that she knew we were there and what we were doing.

What would you say is the lasting legacy June left behind?

June's legacy is that of a loving, caring, and kind person. She was a beautiful person inside and out. Her signature was a warm and radiant smile. She possessed the greatest of all virtues and the least sought after – humbleness. She thought nothing of her own many accomplishments. She was a dedicated servant of the Lord and unselfishly gave of her time and talents for the benefit of others. She will always be my bright star of inspiration. She is loved and missed by all who knew her.

What made you decide to start the website?

I wanted to do something to preserve June's memory and to honor June. I also wanted to do something to promote Alzheimer's awareness, funding for Alzheimer's research and to promote proper care practices. I wanted a site that would be helpful to the families of Alzheimer's victims as a source for up-to-date and reliable information. I wanted a site that would reflect my experiences with this dreaded disease.

I selected a professional site designer and worked with that designer in the design and construction of the site. I wanted a site that was attractive and pleasing to the eye. I wanted a site that was easily navigated. We have many drop down menus. I wanted it to also reflect June's Christian faith. I purchased June's own domain name. I arranged for a site hosting and retained a web site technical person to help me with any malfunctions or additional future changes needed in the site design or operation. The site has been operational since June of 2008.

The Commissioner of the Minnesota Department of Health has told me that June's web site is a "resource for professionals."

Currently there are 180 articles or essays on the site. Last year we had over 100,000 visits to the site by persons from 112 countries. Even places like Syria and Iran and Outer Mongolia are interested in Alzheimer's and visit June's site. The top three countries providing visitors outside the United States are Italy, Spain and Russia. I have had requests to advertise on June's site. These requests have been ignored. June's site is not intended to be commercial in any way.

The address of June's site is: www.junebergalzheimers.com

I have made provisions in my will to have the site operational for at least ten years after I pass on.

Finding My Father

ABOUT THE AUTHOR

Holly Cordova Gaskin grew up on eastern Long Island and now lives in upstate NY with her husband Pieter. Her other books include <u>A Little Company</u>, a thriller/ suspense novel set during the Great Depression, and <u>Tricked</u>, a fast-paced, scary Halloween story for kids. She is also an award-winning radio broadcaster.

www.hollygaskin.com
www.findingmyfather.net

Made in the USA
Charleston, SC
01 November 2014